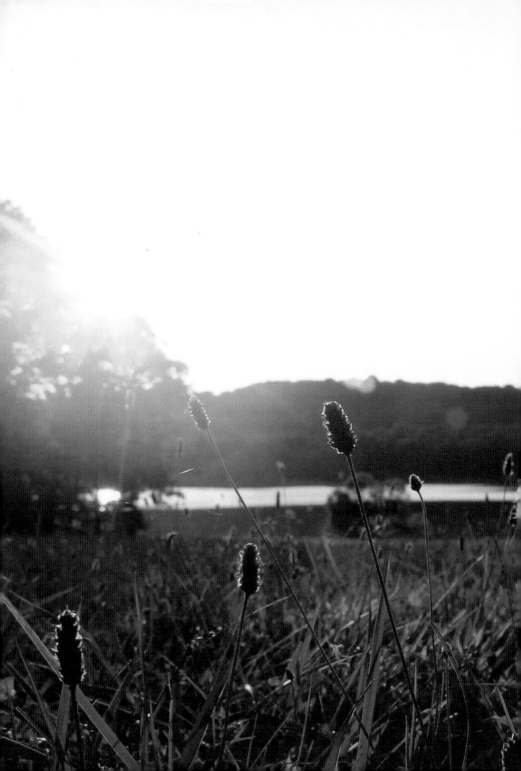

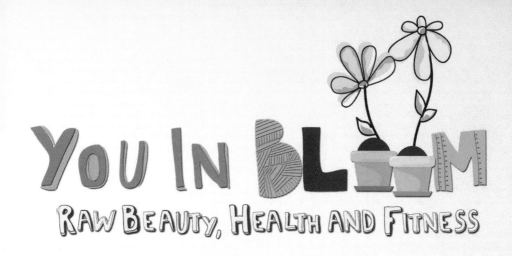

YOU IN BLOOM

RAW BEAUTY, HEALTH AND FITNESS

Megan Elizabeth

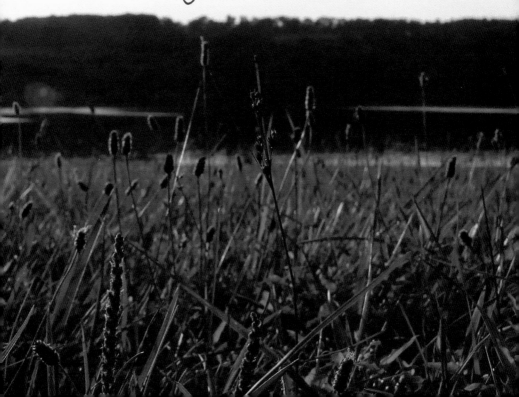

You In Bloom

Raw Beauty, Health and Fitness
Megan Elizabeth

Photography by Joey Borden and Megan Elizabeth
Cover design by Joey Borden and Megan Elizabeth
Edited by Josh Fossgreen, Katie Hayward, Megan Elizabeth, Patricia DeVoy McDonnell, Rich McDonnell and Rally Stanoeva

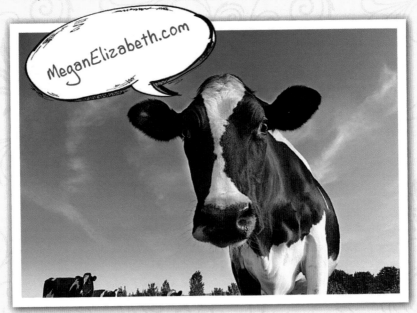

Thank you

Special thanks to my family at Arnold's Way for always encouraging me to live my truth, to Joey Borden for helping me make my ideas a reality, to my YouTube subscribers for supporting me and inspiring me to be creative, and my parents for believing in me.

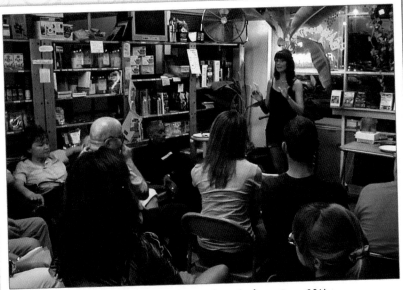

My Second Home (Arnold's Way) – May, 2011

Medical and Exercise Disclaimers

This book is not intended as a substitute for the medical advice of physicians. The reader should regularly consult a physician in matters relating to his or her health and particularly with respect to any symptoms that may require diagnosis or medical attention. The opinions expressed in this book are made by the author only, and the reader takes full responsibility for taking and using the advice provided herein.

The author and publisher advise readers to take full responsibility for their safety and know their limits. Before practicing the skills described in this book, be sure your equipment is well-maintained. Do not take risks beyond your level of experience, aptitude, training and comfort level.

Table of Contents

Introduction - Why I Do What I Do - 2

Part 1: Eating Great - 6
Just Tell Me What To Eat To Make Me Beautiful - 8
How Do I Start Eating More Raw Food? - 11
Where Should Most of My Calories Come From? - 14
Supplements...Why and What? - 18
What I Eat On An Average Day Seasonally - 23
Avoiding Food Fights (Food Combining) - 27
Fun Fruity Facts for Beauty and Health - 30

Part 2: Hey Pretty Lady! Is That Fruit On Your Face? - 38
Homemade Raw Fruit Makeup - 40
Natural Skin Care - 53
Fun In The Sun - 62

Part 3: Everything In Its Place, Including Your Butt - 70
My Fave Five - 72
Pick A Part, Any Part - 75

Part 4: Bonus Recipes - 92
Banana Berry Oatmeal Crumble - 94
Moo-less Chocolate Raspberry Smoothie - 95
Cherry Vanilla Ice Cream Smoothie - 96
Megan's Famous Mango Chutney - 97
Rock'n Ranch Salad - 98
Zucchini Alfredo - 99

Conclusion - Yay! You Made It - 100

Why I Do What I Do...

Eating raw is fun, easy, delicious, and satisfying. It's helped me take control of my life and health. It's so simple to start incorporating raw food into your diet one meal and one day at a time. When you start to notice you have better energy, a more balanced mood, and the aches and ailments are beginning to leave, you'll want to add more and more raw food into your diet to see how great you can feel.

I've been at the bottom and I know what it's like. About 5 years ago, at age 21, I thought I was slowly dying. I was losing my physical health and mental health and was bedridden for most of the day, because my brain was being starved of proper nutrition. I followed my doctors advice and dietary recommendations, but nothing was working. No one could identify what was wrong with me.

I eventually found a holistic M.D. who diagnosed me with adrenal fatigue, leaky gut syndrome, and chemical sensitivity. I imagine it was a combination of poor diet and lifestyle over the years and not any one specific event that caused these issues. No one in the standard medical community even accepts these as real conditions, yet thousands of people are suffering from them and told that there is nothing wrong with them.

I tried many different holistic approaches and incorporated many supplements to heal myself, but nothing made me feel good. The one thing that actually gave me significant improvement right away was eating a raw vegan diet. This gave me a platform to stand on and I began to slowly build my health back.

It's a lot quicker to mess up a room than it is to clean it up. The same goes for our health. I spent so many years not treating my body properly. I had terrible sleeping habits, took antibiotics and prescription drugs, ate cheese like it was my job and drank alcohol as a hobby. Although I feel great now and am enjoying life more than ever I can't even imagine how wonderful I will feel in another 5 years.

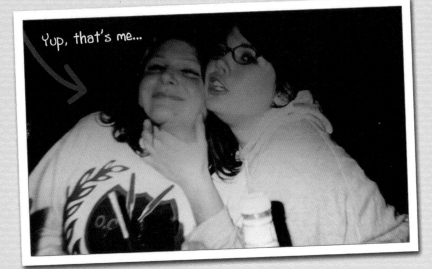

Yup, that's me...

When we fuel ourselves properly we begin functioning at our optimal level. No mid-day crashes, brain fog, or mood swings. No thinking about lunch while you're finishing breakfast. Food becomes delicious fuel and no longer an emotion suppressor or a constant entertainment source.

Food is not the only important factor in health, but it's a big one. One of the problems I found from experiencing chemical sensitivity is that I could no longer use regular products on my skin, hair, and clothes. From years of using toxic chemicals to dye my hair, tan my skin, and make me smell like a field of flowers, my body had reached its tipping point.

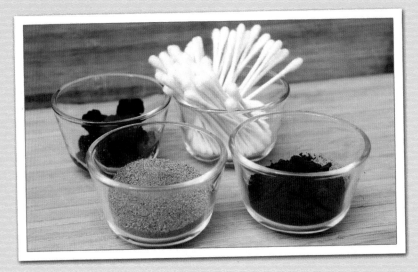

I had to find healthy alternatives to make-up, skin and hair care, laundry detergent and other cleaning products. This stretched my creativity and was actually very fun. Over the past few years I've seen more and more natural products coming onto the market so there's no excuse for using harsh chemicals in your home or on yourself.

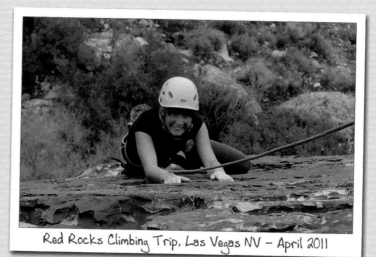

Red Rocks Climbing Trip, Las Vegas NV – April 2011

With all the energy I have now I decided to start putting it to good use. "Fit" was never something I considered myself to be; I just thought I was not meant for such things. I now enjoy exercising by making it a fun activity instead of something I hate doing. I took up rock climbing, running, and love to test my fitness in many different ways. It's amazing how your body can change when you have the right fuel and the right amount of exercise.

The media and advertisements can easily influence people to put all kinds of toxic products and food on and inside their body. Take responsibility for your health and fitness now, because you're worth it and the people who you love are worth it. Eating healthy is a great way to show your love for yourself, your family, mankind, and the planet. Do us all a favor and eat your fruits and veggies like your Mama told you!

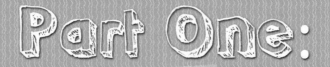

Part One:

Feed Your Face 101

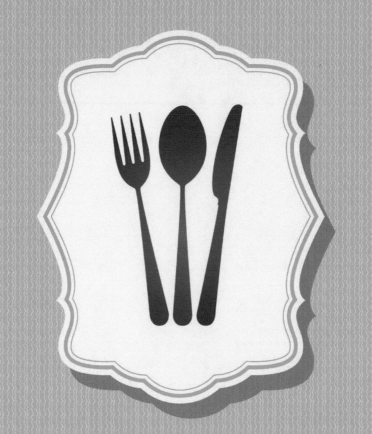

Re-learning How To Eat

There is no one secret food that can change the game for us. It's eating a combination of fruits and vegetables seasonally throughout the year that does the trick. This will ensure you're getting a proper range of fresh and vital nutrients. Taking supplements should only be done when necessary because we can't improve on the amazing package nature has provided for us in raw fruits and veggies. Eating organic is so important too, because it's more nutrient dense and the pesticides used in conventional farming are not good for our bodies. Despite what conventional farmers would like us to believe, pesticides are toxic.

Cancer, heart disease, Alzheimer's, osteoporosis and many other degenerative diseases are on the rise around the world. These illnesses are growing right along with fast food, fried foods, processed foods, and animal product consumption. The more a country increases it's consumption of these so called "foods" the higher illness rates become.

Why has no one in a position of power stepped back and looked at this? I'm sure someone has, but there is way too much money involved to stop this speeding train. Many people are relying on the media and Dr. Oz to tell them what the latest fad supplement is, instead of doing any health research for themselves. Perhaps this is because our society has made health so confusing. There are so many diets! Low-carb, high-carb, high-protein, grapefruit, real food, white food, no white food, the list goes on.

A popular phrase that people are now using is, "Everyone's body is different". I'm not sure what people think they mean when saying this. Is it that we could all do well on a different type of diet? Is it that your liver has a different function than my liver? Do they know what they are saying or are they saying they don't know? Chances are you won't find a fox saying to another fox who is eating a dead rabbit, "well you know, every fox is different, I could never eat a rabbit!".

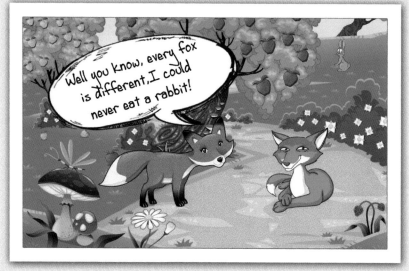

This brings me to my next point. Humans have a species-specific diet, just like foxes, rabbits, horses, gorillas, and so on. We are herbivores by design. Even though we can function on other diets, it doesn't mean they're ideal for us. Don't worry, I'll keep the anatomy and physiology lesson short and sweet. Our canines are small, like the canines of other herbivores, which helps us tear into tough vegetable and fruit matter. We have dull nails that can break fairly easily, not claws that can rip through flesh. We have carbohydrate digesting enzymes in our mouths, which only herbivores possess. We have a long digestive tract that runs on fiber, which is found only in plant based foods, and not in any animal products. We also have an ideal cholesterol number when we consume only plant foods. I'm sure some herbivores occasionally consume bugs or eggs in the wild, but they probably wouldn't prefer them and they're 100% healthy without it. When we eat a wide variety of plant-based foods, we line up almost perfectly with what our nutritional needs are as humans. The exception in my opinion would be certain missing nutrients from our depleted soil and fast conventional growing methods.

Incorporating as much raw food as you can into your daily diet is going to help you have the best possible health. There's not a lot of things in our external world that we can control. There's pollution, worry at work and stress at home. Something we do have control of, however; although many of us like to pretend we don't, is what we put in our mouths.

What we eat is what we are. I figured I better not say "you are what you eat" because that has been said so many times we almost don't hear it anymore. Your body takes what you eat, all the vitamins, minerals, protein, carbohydrates, and fat and is constantly making more of you. More brain, more heart, more love, more happiness, or... more sluggishness, more depression, more wrinkles and more dark circles. What you choose to eat decides what you're going to be contributing to. Do you want to rebuild and restore your body, or do you want to break down and deplete your body?

"Take care of your body. It's the only place you have to live."
— Jim Rohn

How do I eat more raw food?

Eating a raw food diet is easier than you think, because most of us eat raw food already. We just need to increase the amount. I suggest starting one meal at a time. For breakfast, instead of having one banana, try having 6 or more. Huh? You want me to eat 6 bananas? Yeah, I do, here's why:

Say you have 2 cups of oatmeal and you throw in 1 banana, which is a pretty average "healthy" breakfast. That's 395 calories if you just use water and no milk. It's mostly starch, which your body has trouble breaking down and can create skin reactions like eczema or slow down digestion. It requires far more digestive energy than the bananas, pulling energy from the rest of the body. This makes it harder to wake up in the morning and causes lots of people to feel the need for stimulants. Plus, 395 calories is not really enough to keep you full for a long time.

If you focus on calorie restriction when you eat healthy foods, like fruits and veggies you will certainly make up the calories somewhere else. Long before lunch comes you'll being sneaking into the office kitchen to see if anyone's having a birthday today.

Now, maybe your average breakfast looks more like some fluffy yellow stuff and a few salty, crunchy, brown things. If you're eating animal products for breakfast think about this: there's more than 2 full days worth of fat and salt in that one meal. Humans have an ideal cholesterol number when eating an exclusively plant based diet. You're eating a meal that requires the most work to digest. Much of the protein which you would likely eat this meal for becomes denatured in cooking, making it no longer usable. It's also loaded with a bunch of natural hormones from the animal that you're body does not need. According to the Physicians Committee for Responsible Medicine when you eat a diet high in meat and saturated fat you increase your cancer risks by 17%. It may taste good, but not good enough to die for. I don't want to eat something that is going to increase my cancer risks by any percentage.

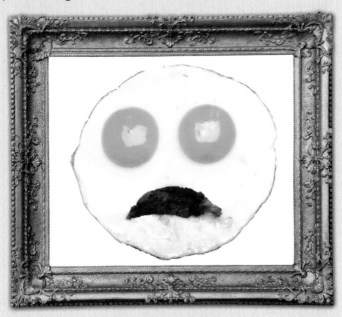

Let's say you had 6 or more bananas for breakfast instead that morning. That would be around 600 plus calories... oh no! "Isn't that too many?", you say. You're going to get your calories from somewhere and it might as well be a healthy food. You'll get over 100% of the Vitamin C you need for the day, it's easy to digest and will last you several hours. You won't feel tired at all and you will eliminate the need to stimulate yourself with coffee and tea.

Here's the point - restricting yourself with healthy foods does you no good. Your body is craving fuel and nutrients and when your blood sugar becomes too low, proper decision making goes out the window. Start one meal, one commitment and one step at a time.

Fruits and vegetables are the two foods that are the highest in vitamins and minerals and are naturally the easiest to digest. Seriously, how can you beat that?

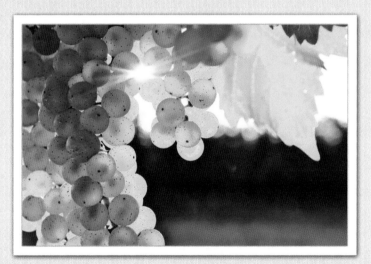

"A fruit is a vegetable with looks and money.
Plus, if you let fruit rot, it turns into wine,
something Brussels sprouts never do."
– P.J. O'Rourke

When starting a raw vegan diet many people are confused about exactly what to eat and when. Later on in this section I will touch on food combining and why it's important to eat foods in proper combinations or alone. Right now though, I want to give you a more general idea of how to eat.

Whole, fresh fruit is the best thing to eat for breakfast because it is quick to digest, contains enough sugar to get us moving, but also has water, fiber, guar and pectin to allow the sugars to be taken up into the blood and cells at a slower pace. Many people forget that most whole fruits are low on the Glycemic Index and are completely healthy even for people with diabetes, as long as they are not eating a high fat diet and processed diet.

In fact, I have many friends who have cleared up hypoglycemia, hyperglycemia, and diabetes through eating a diet high in fruit. Fruits also contain a wide variety of vitamins and minerals and do not need to be fortified like many grain, oat, and corn based cereals and oatmeal. Eat as much fresh fruit as you care for in the morning so that you are satiated until lunch or only need to have a small snack of fruit in between.

Fruit for lunch is also ideal. Lots of people feel a lull in their energy in the afternoon or feel like they want to take a nap after eating lunch. We can prevent this by not causing digestive stress to our bodies. When we eat meals that are heavy on our digestive system it pulls blood flow from the rest of the body to help break down your food. This decreases circulation and makes you feel lethargic or sleepy.

You want to continue to eat vitamin, mineral, and energy rich food throughout the day. Eating light, but incredibly nutritious food in the afternoon is going to help keep your physical energy up as well as your mental energy. My mental energy throughout the day has improved greatly since eating a raw vegan diet.

While working at Arnold's Way Raw Vegan Cafe I got to know and become friends with a great deal of customers. Arnold's biggest seller at the cafe by far is fruit smoothies and green smoothies, which contain mostly fruit. Many people from local offices and businesses come into Arnold's every day for lunch and order giant fruit smoothies. They aren't eating completely raw, but for many of them it's a huge improvement from their former lunch of pizza, sandwiches, and Chinese food. We would hear over and over again from so many customers how having the fruit smoothie kept them alert and satiated for many hours after lunch, compared to what they were having before.

Before dinner I always have another small fruit meal if I'm hungry. I do this because I know it will digest quickly before my dinner, but will help me get in any extra calories I need before eating a big salad. Salads can be incredibly nutrient dense, but they're often not too calorie dense unless you're slathering it in some really unhealthy dressing.

My salad dressing, whether sweet and made of fruit or savory, made with overt fats, such as nuts, seeds, or avocado is usually around 200 to 300 calories. The rest of the salad, even though it's over a pound of lettuce and has other veggies added to it is not more than 75 calories, so I can't expect a salad that has 375 calories maximum to satisfy my hunger if it's calories I'm needing. This is why sometimes people attempting raw diets without any kind of guidance feel hungry all the time and confused as to how people are eating all raw. They are eating vegetables throughout the day and not enough fruit, thus not getting enough calories for their size and activity level.

Fruit is higher in vitamins than minerals and vegetables are higher in minerals than in vitamins. This works out perfectly for us, because as humans we require a large amount of vitamins, especially water soluble ones, like Vitamin C, and smaller amounts of minerals. Eating a diet of mainly fruits throughout the day and lots of greens and vegetables for dinner makes it easy for us to reach the amount of vitamins and minerals we need. We should also incorporate fats in different varieties as well, but this can be done on a more sporadic basis depending on what you're craving.

Your body knows what is in a particular food and it knows what is calorically dense and what isn't. I like to think of my body as having a sort of rolodex, if you will, of what nutrients are in each food that we've eaten before. When we're eating a clean diet that is not full of stimulating and addictive foods, we can actually start to have cravings and develop a taste for certain foods based on what we need nutritionally.

In my opinion, there are certain cases, depending on the quality of the food and the health history of the individual, that may cause the need to supplement some nutrients. Since it could be different for everyone I recommend getting a blood test if you feel you may be lacking something in your diet. For the most part though, when we eat a variety of fruits and vegetables and occasional nuts and seeds throughout the year we get the right range and ratio of all the nutrients we need without making a huge effort and focusing on any one specific nutrient at a time.

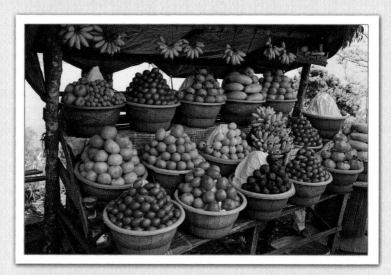

"Variety's the very spice of life, that gives it all it's flavour."
— William Cowper

Supplements... Why and What?

I am not big on supplements myself because I believe that a whole food source of any vitamin is always the best option. A lot of supplement companies today are selling junk. They are loading up their supplements with versions of vitamins that are not even absorbable and usable to us. D2 is the perfect example of this. You find it in many multivitamins, yet D3 is the usable form. No wonder so many people are deficient in Vitamin D despite supplementation.

Currently, the best way to monitor your daily nutrient intake and needs is to input everything you're eating into Cronometer.com. It will help you see the break-down of almost every nutrient you need, plus it will show you your macronutrient ratio of carbohydrates, fat, and protein.

Depending on the amount of variety you're eating throughout the week, you many notice some days you're a little low in one area and then another day you're above the recommended daily amount for the same nutrient. This is fine for most nutrients except water soluble ones, like vitamin C and the B-complex. You want to make sure you get sufficient amounts of these daily. If you're consistently on the lower end for a particular nutrient it's worth investigating to see what raw plant foods may contain it. Google it!

When you see that you're consistently not going to be

able to eat enough quantity of the fruits and veggies you need to meet your daily requirements, this is when you supplement. Regardless of what the reason is, whether you are not able to fit it in or you simply don't want to eat certain foods, in my opinion, this is a case for supplementation. A good example of this would be iron. I have to eat a large amount of leafy greens and certain fruits regularly to get sufficient amounts. Women have higher requirements than men. Some people may say this situation is a cause to venture outside a plant based diet and eat meat, which is high in iron. This is definitely not a good solution.

When we look at other herbivores, like gorillas or horses, their physique tells us that it's quite easy to build muscle on a plant based diet. These creatures spend hours and hours eating and they are also fairly physically active. For almost all herbivores in the wild much of their day is spent consuming plant matter. Most of us can't do this. We have responsibilities that require us to eat smaller condensed meals. Meat and dairy products have taken more precedence in our diet because they are extremely condensed calorie sources and fill us up in our short windows allotted for eating.

This is okay for a little while, but then we start getting all kinds of degenerative diseases, getting sick regularly, and developing allergies. Doesn't this sound like everyone else you know? The benefits of the denser, meat and dairy, do not outweigh the negatives of developing illnesses and dying of heart attacks.

This is why, in my opinion, it is better to seek out a plant food you like containing a nutrient you need or to take a whole food organic supplement of whatever you might be low in, instead of looking for an animal food source, especially if you're in the process of transitioning to a whole fruit and vegetable based diet from a standard diet. You are certainly getting far better nutrition than before, and your body will thank you for that, but if you want to be totally topped off with your nutrients, then definitely look into taking a whole food multivitamin or specific vitamins temporarily until you completely transition to a raw food diet. The best brands I've seen so far are Garden of Life's, Vitamin Code and another similar sounding brand called Source of Life Garden. These whole food vitamins are probably the best ones available right now that I know of.

I've heard the argument that taking a synthetic form of a vitamin is better than the whole food supplement because it truly contains the amount expressed on the label, whereas a whole food supplement may be lacking in potency depending on soil and growing methods. I don't believe this is the case most of the time because scientists are able to measure the quantity of any nutrient in a food. I couldn't locate any studies proving or disproving this, but I imagine that most companies creating whole food supplements would have the food tested to find out about the nutrient content and density.

A few nutrients that I personally supplement to be safe or because I've found benefit from them are:

Vitamin B12 (methylcobalamin form)
Most noticeably it will improve mental clarity and mood in people who are low. You may also notice tingling sensations or numbness in your limbs when you're low in B12. This vitamin should be produced in the intestines by healthy bacteria, but our ability to produce and recycle it within our bodies has been affected by our past health and poor food choices, along with taking antibiotics. It's also possible that some of our B12 needs were met from

eating fresh produce with healthy soil that contained B12 or its cofactors.

Chromium
Contributes to sugar metabolization and will often cause "melon belly" or an acidic feeling when you're low. Chromium is usually found in fertile soil and should be taken up into our vegetables before they're picked. Since our soil isn't as nutrient rich as it once was, due to our modern mono-crop growing methods, it may not contain as much chromium. The biggest problem however is that chromium is one of the last nutrients to be taken up into the soil and most crops are picked slightly early because of the high demand for quick turn over.

Vitamin K2
Contributes to healthy bones and can manifest as dental issues when you're low. Vegetables are very high in K1 and we can easily get sufficient amounts of Vitamin K. K2 however is similar to B12 in that our intestinal bacteria should produce it and we should be able to recycle it within our bodies. I believe that because of our compromised intestinal bacteria, from previous unhealthy diets most of us cannot produce sufficient amounts on our own. The best vegan food source of the vitamin is in fermented foods. I prefer not to eat them regularly so I choose to take a supplement of the vitamin that is produced from fermented vegan foods.

Vitamin D3
I like to keep this supplement handy in case I have prolonged periods without sun. Low levels can cause all kinds of symptoms from mood changes, to low energy, reduced workout recovery, weak bones and teeth, and

many other symptoms. I found a vegan source of the vitamin through the company, Source of Life Garden (not to be confused with Garden of Life whose D3 is not vegan). Your body can store a good amount of Vitamin D in the liver, but usually not enough to last several months. In the winter, if you are not somewhere near the equator getting at least an hour or more of full sun exposure daily, you should have your levels checked and think about supplementing to prevent health issues.

All of the supplements I've listed are currently what I choose to take. As more information becomes available to me and I continue with this diet and lifestyle, these supplements might change.

In an ideal world we would not have to supplement at all when eating our natural diet. I believe raw fruits and vegetables to be the most nutritious food source for humans. In my opinion, if we are not meeting our needs with them, we may not have enough variety in our diet or it may be the result of modern agriculture. The demand for mono-crop farms have depleted our soil terribly and we are not always able to get perfect nutrition because of this. We can only do our best and look for next the best way to find it, which might be supplementation.

I recommend that you check with your doctor about supplementing before you begin if you're unsure what you might need.

To give you an idea of what I might eat on an average day I've shown four different seasonal examples. I definitely eat much more variety than this throughout each season because I snack on lower calorie fruits like apples, berries, kiwis, a variety of melons, pears, peaches as well.

My staples may change to more tropical fruits like cherimoya, mamey sapote, rollinia, sapodillas, and different banana varieties when I'm in a tropical location. There, my snacks might be, lychee, rambutan, and sugar cane.

Use this information as a guide to help you decide how much and what to eat for yourself when you are first starting out. Then as you feel like you're getting the hang of it, you can begin to expand your fruit horizons.

As I said earlier, you want to eat a range of different fruits throughout the year. Having a staple fruit like bananas, that are always available and fairly cheap compared to most fruits, is a good idea. Incorporating other fruits like berries, citrus, figs, melon, and persimmons can be done seasonally.

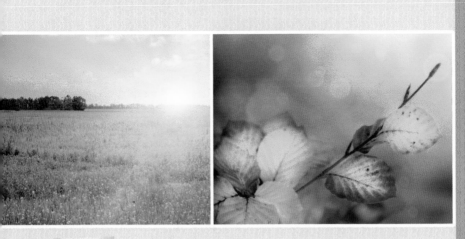

Summer

Breakfast: Half a large round watermelon and 2 to 3 bananas. (Give 30 minutes or more for the watermelon to digest)

Lunch: 6 to 7 bananas in a smoothie with water

Pre-Dinner Fruit Meal: 10 to 20 fresh figs

Dinner: Zucchini pasta made from 3 or 4 zucchinis and a dressing of 1 cup fresh basil, 1 cup fresh mint, 1/2 cup fresh squeezed lemon juice, and 3 dates.

Fall

Breakfast: 6 or 7 fuyu persimmons

Lunch: 5 to 6 mangoes

Pre-Dinner Fruit Meal: 4 to 5 bananas in a smoothie with water

Dinner: A salad of 1lb of romaine and spinach mixed, 1 cup chopped tomatoes, 1/2 cup chopped cucumber. A dressing of 1/4 cup raw hemp seeds blended with 1/2 cup fresh squeezed orange juice, 1/4 cup fresh squeezed lemon juice, 1/2 cup cilantro and 1/4 cup chopped scallions.

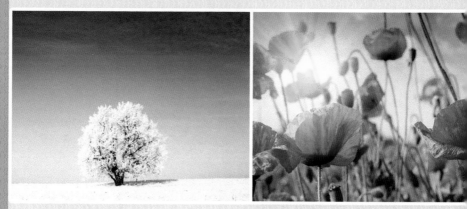

Winter

Breakfast: 8 to 10 juiced oranges (5.5 to 6 cups of juice)

Lunch: 6 to 7 bananas in a smoothie with water

Pre-Dinner Fruit Meal: 8 to 10 juiced oranges

Dinner: A salad of 1lb of romaine and spinach mixed, 1 cup chopped tomatoes, 1/2 cup chopped cucumber. A dressing with 1/3 of an avocado, 3/4 cup fresh orange juice, 1/4 cup lemon juice, 1/4 cup chopped scallions, and 3 to 4 large leaves of fresh sage.

Spring

Breakfast: 10 to 12 juiced oranges (6 to 6.5 cups of juice)

Lunch: 1 to 2 cups of berries blended with 8 to 10 dates (tastes like you're eating pie filling!)

Pre-Dinner Fruit Meal: 4 to 5 bananas in a smoothie with water

Dinner: A salad of 1lb of romaine and dinosaur kale mixed, 1 cup chopped tomatoes, 1/2 cup chopped cucumber. A dressing with 1 or 2 mangoes or 1 1/2 cups chopped mango, 2 dates, 2 large leaves of fresh basil, and 1/4 cup chopped scallions.and 3 to 4 large leaves of fresh sage.

Each sample day comes out to about 2,000 calories. It may be more or less depending on the size of the fruit. Use a calorie calculator when you first start out eating more raw fruits and vegetables to make sure you're getting enough calories for your size and activity level. If you're a guy or if you're a serious athlete you're going to need to eat more than 2,000 calories. Most guys I know eat around 2,500 to 3,500 on an average day and even more when working out.

If you're not a huge fan of mono-meals don't worry! You don't have to eat so simply if you don't want to. This is where food combining comes into play. You can eat different fruit varieties together at one meal if they are combined well.

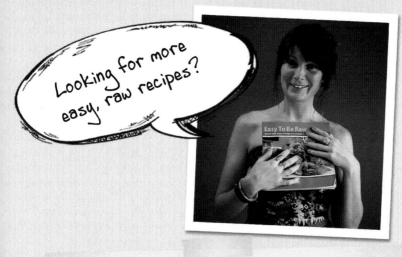

Looking for more easy, raw recipes?

Even though there are some rock'n bonus recipes at the end of this book, check out my first recipe book, Easy To Be Raw, and the add on dessert book to have a full arsenal of low-fat raw vegan recipes under your belt!
www.MeganElizabeth.com/books

I never took food combining too seriously, especially when combining different fruits, until I decided one week to experiment and see if it made a difference for me. I was regularly combining acid fruits like pineapple or citrus with sweets fruits like bananas and dates. I would sometimes get this acidic or "melon belly" feeling in my stomach that would last for 5 or 10 minutes. It was extremely uncomfortable and I had to lay down whenever I felt it. After only a few days of proper food combining I noticed that I had no "melon belly" after fruit meals, everything was digesting perfectly and my skin even seemed smoother and clearer.

I want to explain proper food combining as simply as possible, although it might still seem a little confusing at first. You will get the hang of it though, as I did. It's important to combine what we eat properly so that we can have the best possible digestion and absorption of nutrients.

Just like putting your car into a certain gear for driving at a certain speed, your body digests each food at a certain pace. If you try to go 40 miles an hour in second gear your car is not going to be happy with you. The same goes for your tummy. If you mix an avocado, which can take an hour or more to digest, with a banana, which only needs 30 minutes, your tummy will be angry as the banana starts to ferment. Improper combining leads to a number of symptoms ranging from skin breakouts, to bloating and gas, candida overgrowth, heartburn and also the "melon belly" feeling I was describing before.

The big no-no for raw food combining is mixing fats with sweet tasting fruits at meal time. This is probably the most common combination found in gourmet raw desserts and many standard desserts for that matter. Any sweet fruit, like bananas or dates, or sub-acid fruit, like apples and mangoes, should not combined with overt fats, like nuts, seeds, and avocado regularly. Doing it occasionally is not going to cause ill health and you might not even notice a difference, but if you do it regularly you most likely will feel some symptoms from it.

Combining acid fruits, like citrus or pineapple with fats will digest fine for most people and is okay to combine regularly if you feel you digest it well.

The other bad combo to look out for is making a big party of fruit in your tummy that does not play well together. Sweet fruits like bananas and acid fruits like oranges, just aren't friends and we can't force them to be. They're fine to spend time with separately, but just don't put them in a room together, or rather, don't put them in a smoothie together. Okay, they aren't going to start a fight in a room together, I'm just kidding, but they do not digest well when combined regularly. Like the previous poor combination of sweets and fats, if this combination is done occasionally it should not be a huge deal for most people, but avoid doing it even weekly if you can.

Sweet fruits can be eaten with any other sweet fruits. The same goes for acid fruits, they will digest fine with any other acid fruit.

Sweet fruits include: bananas, fresh dates, sweet grapes, ripe persimmons, sweet cherries, sweet mulberries, and any kind of dried fruit (regardless of it's fresh status as either acid or sub-acid).

Acid fruits include: any kind of citrus, strawberries, pineapple, sour apples, sour plums, cranberries, sour grapes, and pomegranates.

One of my favorite fruits, mangoes, are considered to be a sub-acid fruit. This means they can swing both ways. They can combine well with either acid or sweet fruits in the same meal, but don't think of them as a mutual friend that brings the acid and sweet together. They have to be combined with only one fruit category at a time. So where banana and orange is not a good combo, banana and mango is fine, as well as mango and orange.

A sub-acid fruit can also be eaten with any other sub-acid fruits.

Sub-acid fruits include: apples, pears, peaches, mango, papaya, apricots, cherimoya, fresh figs, cherries, and most berries like blueberries, blackberries, and raspberries, but not strawberries.

Another combination that seems to digest fine for most people is any kind of fruit and leafy greens. I've found that fruit does not combine well with most other vegetables, but a salad with leafy greens, non-sweet fruits, like tomato and cucumber, and a fruit dressing digests great for me and many other raw vegans.

I know this might seem like a lot of information at first, but the more you do it the more it becomes like second nature to you. I'm sorry I just shot down everyone's favorite smoothie combination of banana and strawberry, but you wanted the truth!

Fun, Fruity Facts

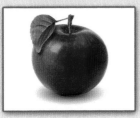

Apples - One of most convenient fruits, I think. They're easy to travel with, available almost everywhere and don't spoil quickly. They're high in B complex vitamins and also contain a good amount of vitamins C and A.

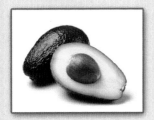

Avocado - A great fruit source of vitamin E. Avocados also contain the carotenoid lutein which promotes eye health. They're one of the more easily digested fats and make a great occasional salad dressing when mixed with lemon or other citrus.

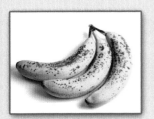

Bananas - Probably the most abundantly consumed fruit by raw fooders and standard eaters alike. They make a great staple calorie source because they taste sweet, they're high in a range of vitamins, are fairly calorie dense and convenient to grab and go!

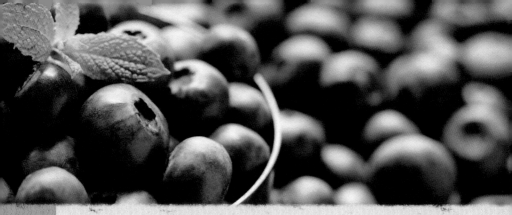

Blueberry - Anti-oxidant rich blueberries are a wonderful addition to any fruit smoothie. They combine well with most other fruits and have a nice thick texture when blended. They also help to enhance dopamine levels in the brain.

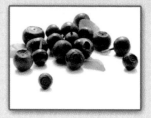

Cherries - This is one of a few fruits that contains anthocyanin in fairly large quantities. It's what makes their color red, but it's also extremely beneficial for those with joint pain and arthritis.

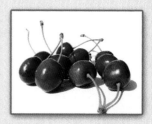

Cucumber - This crunchy green fruit will help you hydrate your body as well as regulate your body temperature and flush out accumulated toxins.

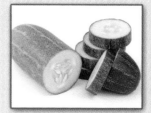

Dates - This fruit probably beats apples for convenience, but they make a great duo together! They're a great calorie source for traveling, and are high in a range of minerals.

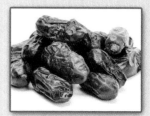

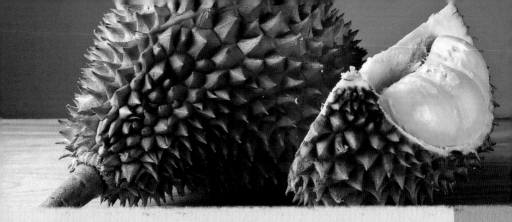

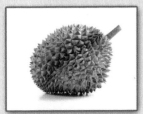

Durian - Some people believe it to be an aphrodisiac. I can say I've seen it make people very happy while they eat it. Because of its sweetness yet higher fat content our body recognizes it as a good fuel source and give us a dopamine release in our brain when we eat it. It has a unique and sometimes acquired taste, but is a great vitamin, mineral and calorie source all around.

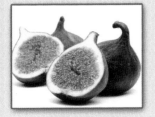

Figs - A very mineral rich fruit, high in calcium, copper, potassium, manganese, iron, selenium, and zinc. Wow! They also contain plenty of fiber and pigment-antioxidants, too.

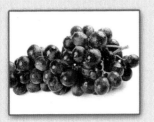

Grapes - A natural source of Resveratrol, which has been shown to have anti-aging effects when consumed regularly. Grapes also contain a wide range of vitamins and minerals that differ slightly in each of the 50 varieties of table grapes.

Honeydew - Contains folic acid, also known as B9, which helps carry proteins to rebuild cells in our body. It's high in vitamin C and very hydrating as well.

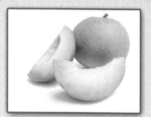

Jackfruit - Helps to strengthen bones, because it's high in magnesium, which is calcium co-factor. This means it helps calcium become more absorbable. It also aids digestion because it's high in fiber. Plus it tastes delicious and it's where they got the flavor for juicy fruit gum!

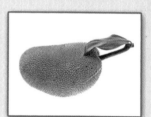

Kiwi - According to Rutgers University it's the most nutrient dense fruit ounce for ounce. One serving contains more than double the amount of vitamin C you need daily!

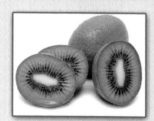

Lemon - Such a versatile fruit. We put it in our water, on our salad, use it as blemish treatment for our skin and can even use it for cleaning. Try adding some to your water in the morning to wake you up and help stimulate digestion.

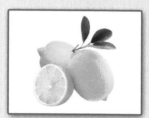

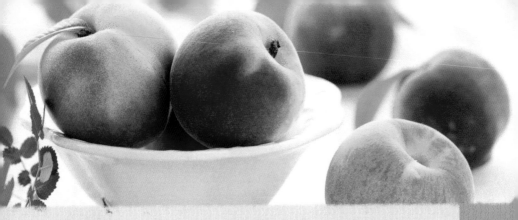

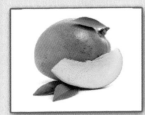

Mango - One of my favorite fruits by far. There are over 500 varieties of mango in the world. Each one tastes different yet still like a mango. They're a great calorie source, averaging around 130 calories each, and they're very high in vitamins C and A.

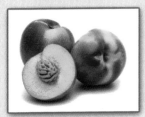

Nectarine - AKA The bald peach. They have a slightly different taste and tend to be more aromatic than peaches. They also contain slightly higher amounts of the same nutrients.

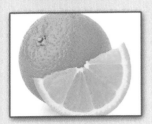

Orange - There are so many different varieties of oranges and surprisingly they are one of the higher protein fruits, containing about 7% of the total calories from protein. My favorite variety is the blood orange, which has a smooth flavor with a hint of cranberry. They're all high in vitamin C as well as A and B-complex vitamins. They travel well and have a longer shelf life than most other fruits.

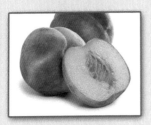

Peach - High in the carotenes lycopene and lutein, they're extremely beneficial for eye health. They're known as the Northern mango because they have a very similar flavor to mangos and belong to the stone fruit family along with almonds, apricots, cherries, mangos, and plums.

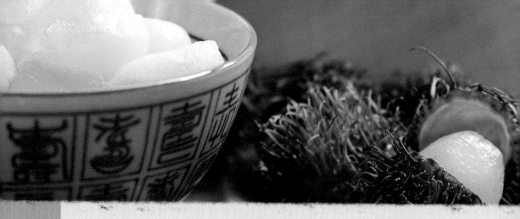

Rambutan - Such a refreshing little burst of flavor. One serving packs a good amount of the RDA of iron as well as tons of vitamin C. They've shown to have anti-parasitic properties and aid in healthy digestion.

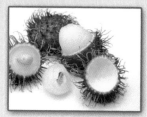

Strawberry - Loaded with powerful antioxidants and anthocyanin, they're very anti-inflammatory. They're the only berry which is considered an acid-fruit and should not be combined with sweet fruits like bananas and dates in large amounts. They go great paired with mangos, oranges, peaches and other berries.

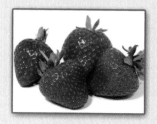

Tangerine - Orange's funky cousin! They're more tart, but have a special flavor that's great when eaten alone or combined in juice with oranges. High in vitamins C and A and offering a good 5% protein.

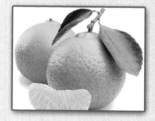

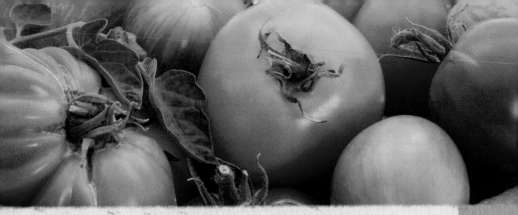

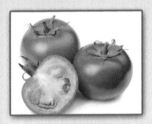

Tomato - One of the best lycopene sources of all the fruits. Tomatoes are also high in potassium and relatively low in sodium, surprisingly. They contain plenty of vitamins A and C and contain a range of other minerals.

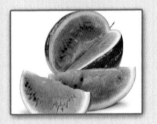

Watermelon - Packing an even higher amounts of lycopene than tomatoes, watermelons are more than just refreshing! They help maintain proper body temperature and keep you hydrated.

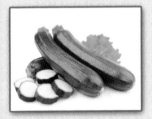

Zucchini - Make a great pasta alternative when spiralized and it's the perfect break from the typical raw food dinner, which is usually a huge salad for me. They're about 16% protein and are loaded with phytonutrients.

For more information on the benefits of
following a raw or plant based diet...

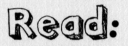

The 80/10/10 Diet by Dr. Douglas Graham

Avoiding Degenerative Disease by Don Bennett, DAS

Easy To Be Raw by Me!

The Engine 2 Diet by Rip Esselstyn

China Study by T. Colin Campbell and Thomas M. Campbell

Raw Revelation E-Book by Dr. T.C. Fry and David Klein

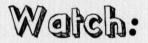

My Weekly Videos at www.YouTube.com/EasyToBeRaw

7 Steps To Staying Young by Arnold Kauffman

Forks Over Knives

Healing Cancer From The Inside Out

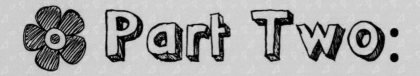

Part Two:

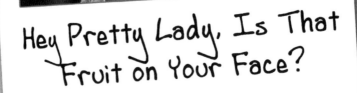

Hey Pretty Lady, Is That Fruit on Your Face?

When I first began my "all natural" lifestyle I was a little sad that I couldn't use all the makeup, lotions, and soaps I loved anymore. It wasn't just a matter of choice, but because I had become chemically sensitive. I went almost a full year without using anything on my body but water and Dr. Bronner's soap.

Then one day it dawned on me that Native Americans and lots of other indigenous cultures would use what they found in nature to make body paints and makeup. So I began experimenting.

The first thing I discovered a few years ago was that beets could be used as cheek and lip color. Since then, I've figured out how to make my own raw eye makeup as well as perfected the cheek and lip color.

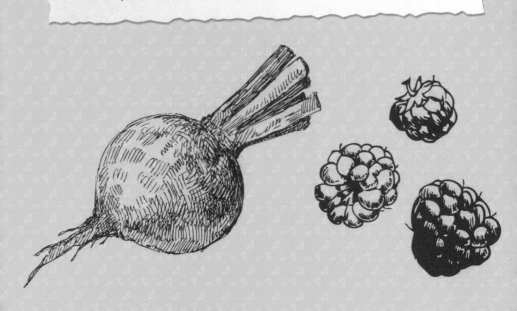

Look mom! I've got fruit on my face! This is one of my favorite things about raw food. I can put it on my face as make-up. If any of the techniques I share below are not for you, later in this section I talk about some alternative options for natural makeup.

List of Tools I Use:

Eyelash Brush
Eyelash Curler
Q-tips or Eye Shadow Applicators

Raw Ingredients You Can Choose From:

Beets - Pink
Frozen Blackberries - Muted Red/Pink
Frozen Raspberries - Bright Red
Activated Charcoal - Black/ Grey
Carob - Light Brown
Cacao - Light/Dark Brown
Spirulina - Dark Green (looks purple, dark brown, or black depending on how much you mix with the berry)

Just a quick word about frozen berries vs. fresh ones; I find that the frozen ones work better as fruit makeup because they're juicier when they thaw out. Fresh ones are okay too, but they are just a little harder to work with. Also it's cheaper to use frozen ones throughout the year because they're really only in season during the summer.

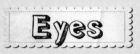

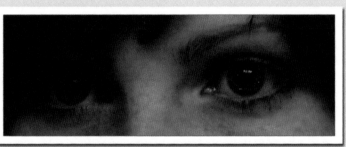

Eyes are the windows to our soul supposedly, so we better hang some nice curtains to entice people to look into them. Not funny? Okay, I won't quit my day job! But seriously, I think it's important for us all to feel confident in our skin.

Some of us feel great without wearing any makeup, but if you're like me, you like to kick it up a notch. I enjoy playing with color on my face in the same way I would enjoy decorating my home, and both are a chance for me to show the world what I can do.

The two ingredients I currently use on my eyes are blackberries and spirulina. Mostly because that's what I happened to have in my house when I started messing around with creating a darker color for around my eyes. Also I felt comfortable with putting those ingredients on my eyes.

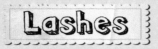

Lashes

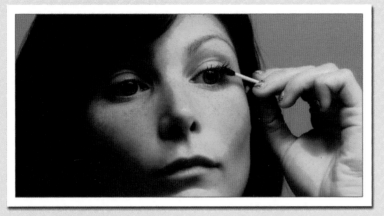

You want this to be mostly berry juice with a bit of spirulina, or carob, cacao, or activated charcoal to add a slight thickness. Choose whatever powder you like.

To apply: Use a Q-tip. Pull about 2/3 of the cotton off of one end and leave the other end alone. This is so you can use one side to apply the color without it soaking up all the juice and the other side for cleaning up anything left behind.

Let your blackberry thaw just slightly. Use the end with less cotton to dip and roll on the slightly frozen blackberry or in its juice. Then just get a little of the powder of your choice on there and roll it on the berry again.

Now you can apply it to your lashes just like mascara. If you need to separate your lashes at all you can use the brush tool.

Let it dry completely. You can add a second coat to make it thicker after it dries. Let your second coat dry completely before you use the eyelash curling tool.

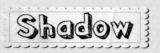

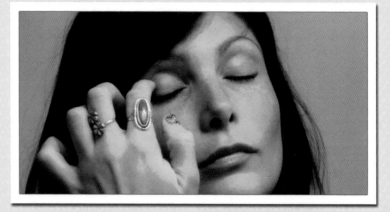

I like to use spirulina and/ or blackberry juice on myself because it has a unique look. You can also use carob, cacao, or activated charcoal powder if you're looking for a more neutral or darker color.

I find that the spirulina and carob don't stick as well as the other colors, possibly because it generally has a courser grind. It sits okay on the outer corner of the eye lid and along the top of the lash line, but doesn't do as well to cover the whole lid.

When I add color with blackberry juice alone I do it above the crease of my eyelid. This is mainly because if you get it in the crease of the lid it can be sticky. Putting it along the top shows the color without causing your lids to feel sticky once it dries.

To apply: Use a new Q-tip, dip it in the berry juice and apply along the crease of the eye or in the desired areas. Sometimes you'll have to do a little smearing with your finger afterwards. It can get a little messy, but everything cleans up easily with a wet Q-tip. You can use the same method to apply other shadow colors. Just dip the Q-tip in the powder and apply to the desired areas.

Using the darker powders like carob, cacao, or activated charcoal will give a much more dramatic look. They tend to be ground more fine and stick to the lid a little better.

In case you're wondering what activated charcoal is: Charcoal is usually made from charred wood that essentially turns into carbon. Then the carbon is treated with oxygen which opens up millions of tiny pores in between the atoms.

You can usually find all these ingredients at your local health food store and they will last you longer than most other forms of makeup since they come in larger quantities. I remember buying new make up all the time before, but now I buy a bag of frozen berries once a month, and I've been using the same spirulina bottle for 2 years!

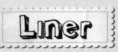

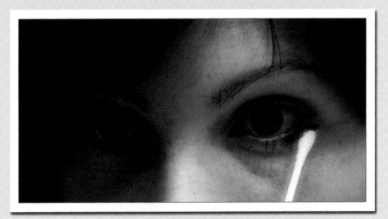

You can use the same or a new q-tip for lining your eyes, or you can even use a regular eye shadow applicator if you have a clean one. You just want it to be able to pick up the powder easily.

To apply: Dip the Q-tip or applicator in the powder. Run the q-tip or applicator along the bottom lash line underneath the eye pressing it in a little as you go to help it stick. You can go the full length of the lashes or just do half of the under eye lid. They both look great and have a different effect on the whole look.

Helpful Tip

Do your best not to get the powder in your eye. It did take me doing it a few times to master the technique. Keep a clean Q-tip handy the first few times until you get the hang of it. Any powder will be absorbed quickly off your eye with the Q-tip.

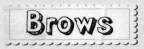

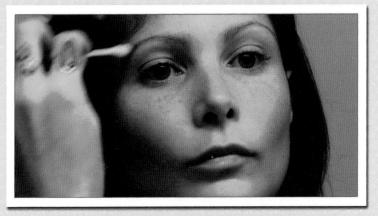

Some of you may have thick and glorious eyebrows... me, not so much. Like many other girls I experimented with changing the size and shape of my eyebrows, even going to the thin penciled-in look at one point. Sadly, they never grew back completely.

Now, I like to fill them in a little bit because having the right shape and thickness can make all the difference in the rest of the look you create. They frame your eyes and balance your whole face.

You want to use the same technique as with the berry mascara, except you don't want it to be as thick and dark. You also want to leave all the cotton on the end of the Q-tip for your eyebrows. After you apply the berry juice and powder of your choice, wipe the Q-tip off on the bowl you're using a few times so that when you apply it to your eyebrows it's not as heavy.

Follow the natural line of the eyebrow and simply fill it in. It doesn't work well for people who do not have any eyebrows. It mainly helps to thicken and darken what you have.

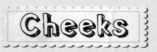

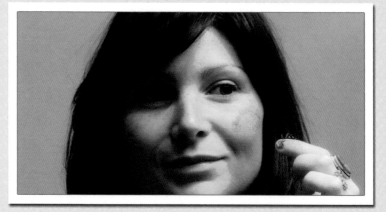

Nothing will add a more youthful look to your face than a bit of blush. Well, except a good facelift... but that's not what we're about here!

There are a few different options for giving your cheeks a rosy glow. Each description is based on how the color appears on my skin, so it may be different for you on your skin.

Beets

Organic beets are relatively cheap and easy to store in the fridge. They will give your cheeks a fresh bright pink color.

To apply: Cut a thin slice of beet and press it to your cheek. Begin rubbing and spreading the color in the desired areas.

Blackberries

They will give your cheeks a deeper more muted reddish-pink color, sometimes with a hint of maroon.

To apply: While the berry is still mostly frozen you can rub it on your cheek and spread the color, or you can wait until it has melted a bit in a dish and then spread the juice on your cheeks.

Raspberries

Use the same method as the blackberries. They produce a reddish-pink on the cheeks.

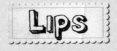

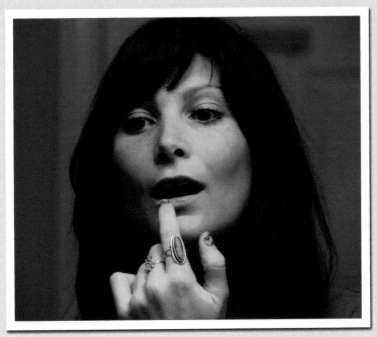

Pucker up! Your boyfriend is going to thank you with kisses for not wearing yucky lipstick!

The options for your lips are the same as for your cheeks. You can use the same color or a different color than you used on your cheeks, because it will turn out totally different either way depending on the color of your lips.

The lip color is the only thing that you would definitely need to reapply, mainly after eating or drinking. Using a beet for your lips is more convenient for taking with you, but it can be done with berries too. If I know I'm going to want to reapply my lip color later, I just bring along my berry that I used that day in a little ziplock baggy. No, it's not as convenient as regular lipstick, but health and beauty are not always the MOST convenient choice available. If you want to do it, you'll make it work and find a way.

Beets
Cut a thin slice of beet and press it to your lip. Begin rubbing and spreading the color on the lips.

Blackberries and Raspberries
Let the berry thaw a little and you can apply the juice with your fingers or a Q-Tip.

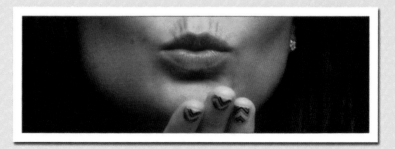

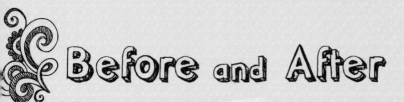

Before and After

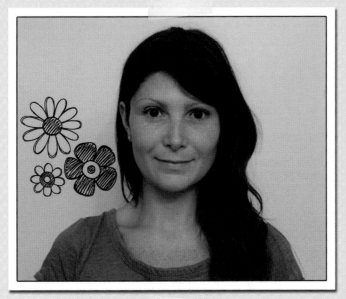

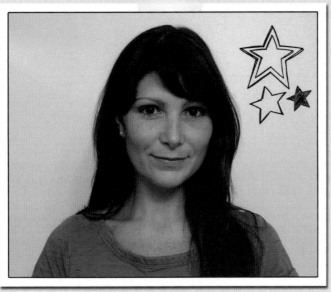

Check out two of my beautiful friends wearing raw fruit makeup!

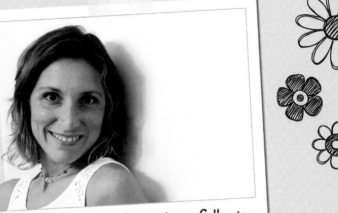

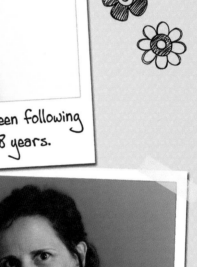

Stephanie is 32 and has been following a raw vegan diet for 8 years.

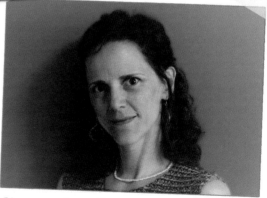

Shaie is 47 and has been eating a high raw vegan diet for the past 3 years

The Next Best Thing to Fruit Makeup

My best makeup recommendation if you feel that raw makeup isn't for you, is using a natural food based makeup brand. The only one that I feel comfortable recommending is the brand, 100% Pure.

They have a fabulous selection of makeup for eyes, cheeks, lips, and skin mostly made from fruit, including some vitamins, herbs and teas, Cacao and Shea butter. Many of their ingredients are organic and vegan, except for a few bee products here and there. They list all their ingredients online in case you want to avoid specific elements or bee products.

People who are extremely caffeine sensitive may not do well with these products because they contain green and black teas, as well as Cacao. Overall though I think many women will enjoy this makeup brand as opposed to their old choice.

They make many body washes, scrubs, and lotions too, that are all natural and have amazing natural scents!

There is also an unprocessed organic raw lip gloss available now called HURRAW. I've tried it and love it. My favorite color is Black Cherry because it looks and smells amazing. It's great to take with you and gives you a beautiful color and gloss.

Check out these products at:
www.MeganElizabeth.com/100pure
www.MeganElizabeth.com/hurraw

Natural Skin Care

Our skin is probably the part of our body that can age us the most if it's not healthy. It is constantly being bombarded with pollutants from the external world and we have to baby it as much as we can to make up for it.

Moisturizing Options

I generally don't apply moisturizer to my skin unless it's necessary and it feels dry, just like I only wash my hair when it's necessary. I try to work with my body and give it some say in the matter, rather than just doing whatever I want to it, whenever I want.

If we wash our skin every day with soap and then apply moisturizer we're just making extra work for ourselves and stressing out our skin. I used to wash and moisturize every morning and night. When I did this, my skin was dry after washing, so I needed to moisturize it. Then later on it would feel a bit oily and I would feel the need to wash it again.

What happens when we wash the natural oils away from our skin and scalp, we just produce more oil. When we rinse with water and lightly dry off with a towel, the oils are not stripped completely, our skin won't feel as dry as it does with soap and we won't feel the need to moisturize as often. Our bodies know how to naturally keep our skin moist and will stop over producing oil within a week or so, sometimes less, if we stop washing it regularly.

The best option if you want to clean your skin regularly is to use just plain water with a washcloth to lightly remove any dirt or sweat from your skin. This will also help to remove any dry and dead skin from the surface.

Sometimes outside influences like chlorine in the water or dry heat can cause dryness. This seems to happen for me mainly on my arms and legs, especially when I'm living in Arizona. I do have an Aquasana carbon shower filter, which helps remove a lot of chlorine, but sometimes it still doesn't make a difference. Shaving can also cause us to be more dry in certain areas. In these cases I consider it acceptable to use a moisturizer, because having dry skin is not good and leads to cracking and diminished skin cell repair.

Below are a few different types of all natural moisturizers I have used and enjoyed. They range from providing light to heavy moisture.

Pear

The idea for using pear as a moisturizer came from Arnold Kauffman. I'm not sure where he got the idea, but he's always trying to make fruit as multi-purposeful as he can. Many times he suggested putting pear on my skin and I dismissed it thinking it would definitely be a sticky mess. Then one day I had no other option and all I had around was a pear, so I gave in and used it to moisturize my legs. It actually worked quite well and was not sticky at all! I was shocked. There was a slight bit of residue which brushed off easily once it was dry.

Simply cut the the pair in half or just cut off a small piece depending on how large the area is you're moisturizing. You can keep the rest in a small plastic bag or some other type of container and store it in the fridge for later.

Aloe

I have an organic aloe plant of my own, which I use small pieces from. I tend to stick with one leaf at a time. The plant continues to grow new shoots in the middle as I use the outer leaves. If you don't have your own aloe plant then you can find large leaves of aloe at Asian markets and store them in your fridge.

I prefer using it straight from the plant because it's very hard to come across packaged aloe that doesn't contain preservatives, even if the aloe itself is organic.

I mainly use this to moisturize around my eyes and anywhere else wrinkles would be likely to develop. Aloe contains a large range of amino acids, many vitamins including A, B complex, C, and E. It's also high in antioxidants like all fruits and veggies. When I apply it regularly I notice my eyes appear more smooth and awake. This is the one scenario in which I feel that moisturizing regularly, even when my skin is not dry, has more benefits than negatives.

If I moisturize the rest of my face this is typically what I use because it helps with dryness without being oily at all. It does have a bit of a tightening effect and I consider it my natural anti-aging and tightening cream.

I just pull off small pieces at a time and open them up to expose the gel inside. Then I rub the gel on my skin, sometimes directly with the leaf and sometimes putting a bit on my finger.

Tate's Miracle Conditioner

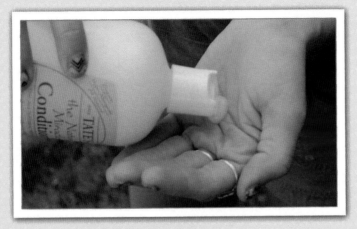

You'll find that Tate's conditioner is a multi-purpose product; the two most popular uses are conditioning hair and moisturizing skin. It has a very light fragrance which comes from the combination of all natural ingredients. They are basically all food based, most of which are grown organically, but not always certified. Being a chemically sensitive person, I can tell when something is not organic and I've had no issues with this product. I love it because it provides the perfect amount of conditioning for hair and skin.

You can apply it generously because a lot of it will absorb quickly and it dries fast. It leaves your skin very smooth and silky. I generally use it when I'm out of the house or on trips because it's easier to take with me and it's not messy at all.

It is a little expensive so I usually call the company directly to order and ask what sales they have going on. I end up buying it in bulk because it's cheaper and I know I'll use it eventually, either as a moisturizer or hair conditioner.

Dr. Bronner's Moisturizing Lotion

This is a more recent product that I had the delight to sample at Whole Foods. There are about four different scent options, made with all natural and organic fragrance of course.

It's a really great product with clean ingredients. It provides slightly more moisture than Tate's Moisturizer, in case you have extra dry skin. It still feels light and is not greasy at all.

I've only seen it recently in a few Whole Foods stores so if you can't find it there you can order it from www.DrBronner.com.

Coconut Oil

Some people absolutely swear by coconut oil and use it religiously. It's a little too greasy feeling for me personally to use regularly. In the winter if my skin is super dry and nothing else works then coconut oil is my last resort. It's just a little heavy and can stain your clothing if you're not careful, but it does a great job of moisturizing and you'll smell delicious!

If you ever get sunburned and need to sooth the area, coconut oil works best. Aloe is great if you have a little pinkness from the sun, but coconut oil will really help a serious sun burn feel better and heal faster. You should always try to prevent burns from happening at all by being in the sun for an appropriate amount of time for your skin and slowly building a base tan, but coconut oil is a great help if you do happen to get burned.

I've seen it available as raw and heated. I prefer to use the organic unheated kind of whatever brand I find on sale from my local health food store.

Cleaning Your Skin

Many of us have gotten into the habit of washing our faces with soap. Like I explained in the moisturizing section above, when we wash our skin constantly it can feel dry, causing us to need to moisturize. Then our skin still wants to make up for the natural oils that were stripped so it produces more oil. Now you have oil and moisturizer on your skin, so you have to wash it again.

If you must wash your skin definitely look for the most natural soap available to you. I use Dr. Bronner's Peppermint soap if I feel I must wash my face. They also have an even milder soap with fewer ingredients made for babies that comes in a bar and a liquid soap.

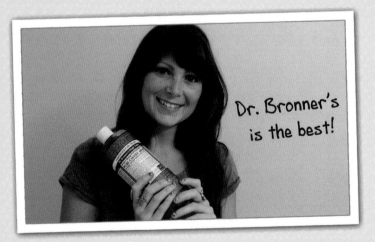

Dr. Bronner's is the best!

I make an effort to only wash the necessary parts of my body in the shower because lathering your entire body with soap will remove Vitamin D from your skin. When we expose our skin to the sun, UV rays actually clean our skin so there's no need to lather up all over unless you're actually covered in dirt.

If you're someone who suffers from breakouts and this makes you want to wash your skin more often, consider using a blend of essential oils or extracts that promote clear healthy skin. The best product I've found for this is called Acne/Pimple Control by the brand, Forces of Nature. They usually sell it at Whole Foods or you can order it online. It will cost you about $25 dollars for a small bottle, but it does work and it will last you at least a month or more. This same brand also makes a great scar treatment that has worked extremely well for me and helps for dry patches and eczema.

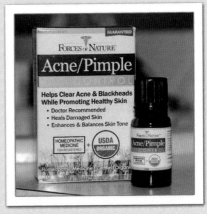

Improving Your Skin's Appearance

Often in the past when I was having a skin issue I would immediately raid my bathroom cabinets for whatever creams and cleansers I could find, or I'd run out to the convenience store to buy some new product that promised to give me perfectly clear, beautiful skin. This usually did not help the problem, but it didn't stop me from trying.

Having clear smooth skin is so much more than what your cleanser, cream, or lotion is all about. It comes from the inside and for most people it's a good refection of what's going on in your body. Some people can eat whatever they want and have great skin, their health might suffer in another area, but for many people their diet and lifestyle effects their skin's appearance more than they can imagine.

Food

What we put into our bodies for fuel makes a huge difference in our skins appearance. The closer I eat foods that I know are ideal for me, the better the appearance of my skin. Sometimes I have to make compromises when traveling. I eat a lot more dried fruits and dates or pasteurized juices. It's definitely noticeable to me by the end of my travels because my skin looks much dryer and is not as smooth. This is most likely due to the fact that I'm not as hydrated, even though I'm drinking plenty of water, as fruits and vegetables contain the most pure and hydrating water.

When I eat low-fat, around the equivalent of 1 avocado a week, keep low-water fruits like dates or dried fruits to a minimum, and drink as much water as I'm thirsty for, my skin is significantly more clear and smooth.

Exercise

Exercising regularly can also improve your skins appearance. Our Lymphatic System plays a big role in detoxification and it relies completely on the movement of our body to circulate the lymph fluid. If we are sedentary our lymph fluid remains stagnant. This can reduce your immune function, make you feel tired, and even cause skin breakouts. Our bodies can detoxify much more efficiently when we're consistently active.

Sleep

Many of us don't sleep enough or at the right times. We figure out the amount of sleep we can get by with and stick to that. Truthfully though, how many of you sleep right through your alarm? Or do wake up to your alarm and think, "I wish I could sleep another hour or two"? Chances are you need more sleep.

Sleep is not just rest from the day's activities, it's meant to be a time of repairing and restoring. The earlier you go to sleep the more restorative it will be. According to many Naturopathic and Holistic Doctors, your body begins its detoxification and repair processes at 10PM. If we're not asleep around that time we might not be as well rested as we could be.

If I'm lacking sleep or consistently going to bed too late, I just don't feel as good. I don't look as great either. When I'm getting tip-top sleep and going to bed on time, I feel and look so much healthier and my skin can glow.

Exfoliating

The easiest and most gentle way I have found to exfoliate my skin is using water and a wash cloth. My skin always appears more fresh and smooth when I do this regularly. Our pores can get clogged with dirt and dead dry skin just loves to hang around. Exfoliating is the best way to get rid of these issues and help your new smooth skin shine through.

Avoid exfoliating daily because it does remove a larger amount of oil than just rinsing with water. Doing it weekly is probably best for most people.

Fun In The Sun

Be Afraid... Be Very Afraid

The American Academy of Dermatology on their website, www.ADD.org, will tell you that there is no safe amount of unprotected UV exposure that will allow for vitamin D production, without increasing the risk of skin cancer. This is scary! We basically should never go in the sun if we want to avoid possibly getting skin cancer, right? Sounds like a great suggestion considering how important the sun is in the function of the majority of living things on the Earth's land, but let's just write it off. We should all move to Norway for the Winter darkness and we can be outside as much as we want without the fear of getting skin cancer. I'll start investing in Vitamin D supplements now!

The misinformation on sun exposure being fed to people today by groups like this and through the media is really sad. A lot of people are terrified of getting skin cancer, but don't educate themselves enough to learn what factors really contribute to it.

How did skin cancer rates jump from about 7 people out of every 100,000 in the 1970's, when barely anyone wore sunscreen, to 36 out of 100,000 in 2010? Is it because of the ozone layer? No, I don't think so, because people are told to avoid the sun and are spending much less time in the sun today than they were in the '70's. Is this because we've produced a generation of less sun resistant people? Well, yes, in a way.

People are lathering themselves in sun screen because they think this helps them avoid skin cancer and burns. This not only interferes with Vitamin D production and absorption, but keeps them pale with no natural resistance to the sun. It makes you much more likely to burn if you're caught without sunscreen and burning increases your skin cancer risks.

Some of the ingredients used in many common sunscreens have recently been studied and the results are alarming. They suggest that oxybenzone, benzophenone, octocrylene or octyl methoxycinnamate (yeah, I can't really pronounce them all either) have been linked to contributing to the most rare, but serious form of skin cancer, Melanoma. So the very lotion that is supposed to prevent skin cancer could be contributing to it? Yes! That must sound crazy to the average person, but to me, the idea of putting chemicals all over your skin and expecting it to help you sounds crazy.

My Mom is 100% Irish, has freckly skin, and did have skin cancer in the past. She spent most of her life avoiding the sun and putting on sunscreen. Somehow though in her late 30's she was diagnosed with skin cancer. She had it removed and everything was fine, thank gosh, but the placement of the cancer was very interesting... it was on the left side of her face, her left shoulder, and left arm. She was a home care nurse at the time and was driving for much of her day.

In the United States and other countries where people drive on the right side of the road, skin cancer is more prevalent on the left side of the body. It's more prevalent on the right side of the body in the United

Kingdom and other countries who drive on the left side.

My Mom was always wearing sunscreen and trying to slather it on me too! So how did she manage to get skin cancer anyway? Many sunscreens only block UVB rays, which can cause sun burn, but they don't block UVA rays, which penetrate more deeply into the skin and cause more permanent damage like wrinkles, sun spots, and skin cancer. Car windows do the same thing, as well as other types of glass.

My mom is no longer a home care nurse, but she can still drive up to several hours a day regularly commuting to work and visiting her parents who live an hour away. She has not had anymore bouts with skin cancer since then, even though her risk factors, like age and sun exposure have increased. She has built up a base tan and no longer frets about sun exposure like before.

She also reduced her dairy and meat consumption, and increased her raw fruit and vegetable intake. She's now 54, cancer free and beautiful as always!

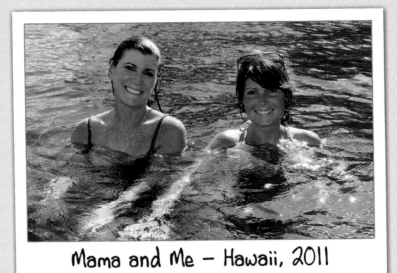

Mama and Me – Hawaii, 2011

People Most At Risk For Skin Cancer

For the most part, the people who are most likely to get skin cancer are those who have avoided the sun and do not build any base tan to protect them from getting burned. Cancer, whether it's on your skin or in your body will thrive in acidic conditions due to poor diets, consisting of meat, fish, dairy and eggs, unhealthy habits like smoking and drinking, and unhealthy lifestyles that lack proper exercise, rest and relaxation. When you eat an alkaline diet of fruits and vegetables and give yourself the amount of exercise and rest you need, your body becomes more alkaline, and cancer does not thrive in an alkaline body.

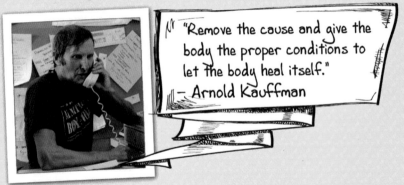

"Remove the cause and give the body the proper conditions to let the body heal itself."
— Arnold Kauffman

After working with Arnold Kauffman at Arnold's Way, I saw this information proven over and over: breast cancer, colon cancer, skin cancer, diabetes, colitis, heart disease, all reversing. What were these people doing? Simply changing to a plant based and mostly raw diet, cutting out habits that stress the body and incorporating new healthy habits.

I Should Go In The Sun Then

Yes! Get out there! Go bask in the golden rays and feel the warmth penetrating your skin! Honestly, doesn't the sun make you happy? When it has been cloudy for days and your mood is just awful, you bump into Sally at work and don't even say excuse me because you're so grumpy. Then, the sun comes out and you feel optimistic! It makes you want to eat your lunch outside and say hello to the guy in your office who always farts, who you never say hello to.

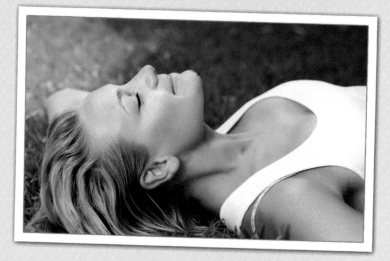

We're designed to be in the sun because that's the way we're supposed to get our Vitamin D in nature, just like we're meant to get all of our nutrients from nature. There are situations that might cause you to need to supplement depending on where you live. Most people, unless you live fairly close to the equator, cannot get enough Vitamin D in the Winter.

I cannot make a specific suggestion for you as to

whether you should take a supplement or not, but if you're worried you might be low you should check with your doctor about testing. I can however, recommend a supplement that is appropriate for those who would like to supplement. Source of Life Garden makes a truly vegan D3 supplement as opposed to most other brands, which source their D3 from lanolin found in sheep wool. There's no way to know if the wool was collected from a humane facility so there's no reason to use it if you don't have to. Taking D3, not D2, is what we want to do if we are not getting sufficient amounts of UVB. Most doctors don't inform their patients of this and many people end up taking D2 supplements instead of D3, which is not usable to us.

On a side note, osteoporosis is a big problem for many people in this country. Vitamin D is crucial for calcium absorption and strong bones. Many standard eaters think drinking cow's milk is helping us with this problem because it contains calcium and is often fortified with Vitamin D. The first problem here is someone would have to drink more than double the amount recommended to reach the minimum requirements of D. The second problem with this is that drinking milk, eating dairy, and consuming animal products in general causes our body's blood and urine to become more acidic. This is common knowledge to most vegans, but not to most vegetarians or standard eaters. To neutralize this acidity our body leaches calcium from our bones. This is why, looking at statistics, we can see the countries that consume the most dairy and other animal products also have the highest rates of osteoporosis, among other degenerative diseases.

Absorbing Vitamin D

The process of absorbing Vitamin D through our skin is more involved than most people realize and it can be easily disturbed. Being exposed to sunlight alone is not enough to produce and absorb it.

One of the main causes of us not absorbing enough Vitamin D as a society is our love for soap and body wash. Rinsing our skin with water does not wash away Vitamin D, but washing your skin with soap does. This is because it's a fat soluble vitamin and not water soluble. Soaps contain fats which easily pick up the unabsorbed Vitamin D.

If you're lighter skinned and you just laid outside during the summer for 30 minutes, 15 minutes on each side, you would have some pretty awesome Vitamin D action going on. Then you might feel kind of sweaty so you take a shower right after you're done. Most people will reach for their favorite body wash, or bar of soap and lather up. Now you're feeling "zestfully clean" but you also just washed off most of your Vitamin D. At least you still have a tan!

Another cause is our fear of the sun, like I talked about earlier, and our need to cover ourselves with sunscreen. Sunscreens, even as low as 8 SPF block our ability to absorb D. Most sunscreens have an SPF of 15 or often higher.

You would think your children who played at the beach all day would have plenty of Vitamin D to spare, but alas they do not because you slathered them in SPF 30. I can absolutely understand wanting to protect your children from being burned. It might be best to help them slowly build the protection of a tan before long periods of sun exposure. This will help them to avoid burns while also absorbing the D they need.

For us to obtain proper amounts of Vitamin D during the summer most fair skinned people need only 5 to 10 minutes on each side of the body daily. Try to expose as much skin as possible. The darker your skin tone, the longer you need to be in the sun to absorb the right amount of D for you. If you have very dark skin you may need to spend 30 minutes or more on each side daily.

Vitamin D is a fat soluble vitamin that doesn't need to be replaced daily because we can store it. This means you could be in the sun for a longer period one day and not need to lay out the next day.

As I said before, in the winter it's almost impossible to get enough if you're not in a place near the equator, so look into getting your levels checked if you think you might be deficient.

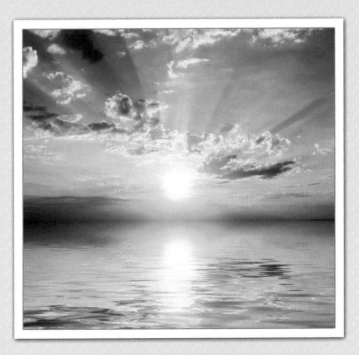

Part Three:
Everything In Its Place, Including Your Butt

The workouts I've included here are meant to give you an idea of what I like to do to stay in shape. After losing 50 lbs. over the course of several years and then becoming so sick and lethargic, I lost a lot of my muscle tone. I've spent the last few years getting my body back into shape so I can feel healthy and strong. Hopefully these workout examples can help you build a workout based on what you need to focus on. Consulting your doctor and a personal trainer is recommended before beginning a new workout routine.

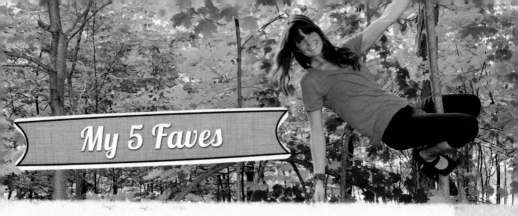

Running

One of my favorite quick workouts is running. If I don't have a lot of time to spare that day and I need a quick pick me up, running a mile as fast as I can does the trick.

Low-intensity workouts do not usually help us get the results we're looking for. We might be burning slightly more calories than when we're not working out, but it's not helping us build muscle, get toned, or really increase our metabolism. I am not by any means into body building or looking extremely muscular myself, but I like to look toned and feel strong.

When we workout at a high-intensity we are producing more lactic acid in our muscles. When we produce lactic acid we are in anaerobic training mode. This helps with building muscle and increasing the metabolism because we're producing more Human Growth Hormone (HGH). HGH enhances cellular repair and helps to slow down aging, burn fat, repair muscle, and regulate the metabolism.

Jumping

If I'm not in a running mood, but I need to get my blood pumping, I might jump on my rebounder for 5 minutes or more. Doing jumping jacks can have a similar effect if you don't own a rebounder.

Doing jumping jacks might not sound like hard work, but try doing them for 5 minutes without a break. It's very challenging at first!

Jumping and really moving your body and all its parts is necessary for healthy detoxification. Our Lymphatic system, which helps clean out unwanted toxins, does not flow like our blood. It only moves with the movement of our body. That's why it's so important to have some sort or activity every day.

Climbing

Rock climbing is one of my favorite workouts. Sometimes I only have an hour to climb at the local gym but that's plenty of time to kick my butt if I climb hard. Ideally I would be in there for 2 hours or more, but it's hard to always schedule that in.

Any type of climbing or exercise that mimics it is great for your body. It's cool to be able to lift up your own body weight, but it's also really great exercise. Doing pull ups or using a pull down bar can help you exercise the same muscles.

Rock climbing incorporates core muscles and leg muscles as well so it's more of a total body workout. I would recommend it to any active healthy person who's looking for a fun time that challenges your mind and body. Climbing trees is also beneficial if you do not have access to a rock gym and you're confident you can do it safely.

Hold That Pose

I love to choose a yoga pose or even just get in plank position on my forearms and hold it for as long as I can. Plank position is similar to that of a push up except you're holding yourself up with you forearms instead of your hands. One of the best ways to build muscle is pushing them until failure.

When I first started out holding a forearm plank I could only hold it for about 1 minute and 30 seconds. Currently my best time is 3 minutes and 30 seconds and I'm confident it will keep improving slowly. My stomach muscles, lower back muscles, and triceps are where I feel it the most when holding this position and have noticed they're much stronger now.

The Dreaded Pushups

I don't know too many people who just love pushups, even if they do them regularly. They are, however; extremely effective for toning many muscle groups. The main muscles you're working are your pectorals and triceps, but if you're doing a perfect pushup and holding a nice straight line then you are working your legs and core as well.

If you can't do a perfect pushup just yet then start out on your knees. It's more important that your back is straight and firm and hands are in the right position, which would be a couple inches outside of being just under your shoulders. Touch your chest to the ground and keep your core nice and straight as you come up, don't let your back sag in. Do as many as you can until you simply can't do another! I suggest doing them 3 or 4 days a week.

After a couple weeks you can switch to doing regular pushups. You might be doing a lot less at first, but you will be getting an even better workout as long as you keep proper form.

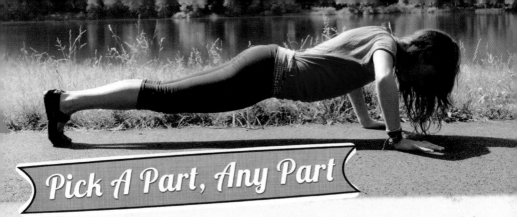

Pick A Part, Any Part

Working out at a gym, using free weights and doing abdominal exercises is not what I used to think of as fun. It took a while for me to figure out how to mentally enjoy my work outs and get excited for them. I figured out a way for me to get the best results in the shortest amount of time. I do not do any set amount of reps and I do not do sets. I do each exercise once and take myself to the limit. If I do each of these exercises below pushing myself to failure, instead of stopping and starting a new set, I find that I build muscle better and burn more fat.

Don't You Love Ab Workouts? Not!

I've found, as I'm sure many of you have, that I hate doing regular sit-ups. For me, the results of this exercise have never outweighed the negatives. Also if you have a history of neck issues like me then you know how much they can hurt you if not done absolutely perfectly. That being said, I happily try every other abdominal toning exercise I come across.

Forearm Plank

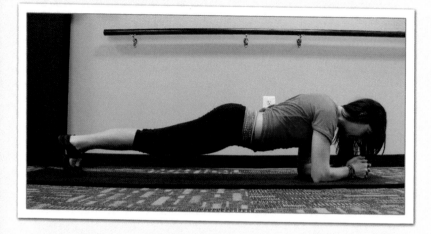

One of my favorites I already shared with you earlier, is holding a plank position on my forearms. This exercise really helps with strengthening your deepest abdominal muscles: the Transverus Abdominis. They're most responsible for holding good posture and are the basis for building good core strength. Forearm plank helps to strengthen all your other abdominal muscles as well as your lower back. You will also feel it in your biceps and triceps, but it won't necessarily build muscle in your arms. You may even feel it in your legs a bit too.

Start out at 30 seconds if that's all you can do and work your way up, trying to add 15 to 30 seconds at a time to your previous maximum time. You might eventually reach a point where you hit a temporary plateau in time, but you will still be getting an amazing ab workout.

Callanetics Waist, Hip, and Butt

The next ab workout I do regularly I learned from a Callanetics tape my Mom had when I was younger. This was one particular exercise that stuck with me from the tape. It tones the side of your waist along with your hips, gluteal muscles, and your hamstrings. Although the full workout was amazing and did give great results, I found that like many types of yoga, it was a little too slow moving for me. I still do some of the other Callanetics exercises, just more sporadically than this one.

You can sit on a yoga mat or a very thin cushion. Pull up a chair next to you or use a low coffee table. Lean on one hip and using the chair or coffee table lightly support yourself by holding on with your 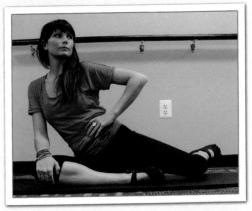 hands. Bend your leg that is closest to the ground in a way that will help you support your body the most. Lift your top leg several inches from the ground and bend your knee slightly. Keep your raised foot pointed and angled slightly up if you can. Once you get into this position you want to move your top leg back and forth only 2 inches at a time. Aim for doing this movement 100 times or a long as you're able to.

Abdominal Twist

Another ab workout you'll always catch me doing in my routine is a sitting ab twist with a medicine ball or light free weights, usually weighing around 5 to 8 lbs. This exercise can also be done with a sit up incorporated in between twists, but I choose not to do that. I find if I do this exercise on its own to failure I really feel it. It's not nearly as awkward for me as sit-ups and your neck is not strained at all.

Find something to anchor the tops of your feet on. You can use a couch or end table to stick your feet underneath. Scoot yourself up so your legs are bent at about a 90 degree angle. Lean back a bit until you feel a slight strain on your abs. Then slowly turn from side to side touching both hands to the ground on each side. Stretch your arms out as far as is comfortable while still keeping your torso straight, leaning to one side as little as possible with your turns. Start out without weights or a ball if you're just beginning with ab workouts, then increase the weight slowly after you feel stronger.

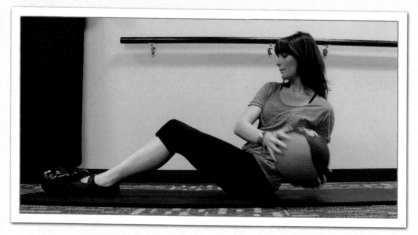

Feel'n The Burn In Your Butt

After I turned 24, I realized I was going to need to make an effort if I wanted to keep my butt in the same place. Doing yoga and using exercise bands didn't cut it for me, I didn't feel the burn enough in my butt, so I've experimented with different exercises to find the most effective ones in my eyes.

Recumbent Exercise Bike

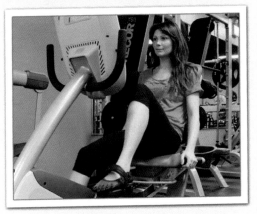

I would typically run on the treadmill in the gym at my apartment complex when it was too hot outside in Phoenix, Arizona. There was almost never anyone in there, which I loved. One day however, my own private gym was occupied and someone was on my treadmill! Running is usually my favorite way to start out my workout routine. I just run a mile as fast as I can. I decided to bike, which I barely ever do and I chose the recumbent exercise bike, because the other one felt uncomfortable. This is the kind of bike where you're sitting lower to the ground. I was thinking, "This is going to be a breeze. How am I going to get a hard workout on this thing?". I'm practically yawning just thinking about it.

I decided I would do 2 miles as hard and as fast as I could on a high setting to try to make up for my lack of running. I huffed and puffed and managed to finish it in around six minutes and 45 seconds. I don't know if that's a great time, but it was surprisingly incredibly hard.

By the time I finished the rest of my workout my butt was so sore! My hamstrings, hips, and quads were also feeling it a bit, too. Then, I had to walk up the stairs to my apartment, wow! I was amazed that I was still a little sore the next day as well. This usually doesn't happen to me unless I'm working completely new muscle groups. I always thought I was getting a good workout just doing leg lifts and squats, but apparently I was barely hitting these muscles at all. Now I try to incorporate biking on a recumbent bike at least once or twice a week in place of or in addition to running.

Try incorporating it into your workout regularly if you're trying to tone up your butt or keep it in place. I find that I get better results when I do shorter spurts of high intensity as opposed to dragging the time out and going slow. Start out with a half mile at a time if you have to, but give it your all and push yourself.

Leg Lifts and Squats

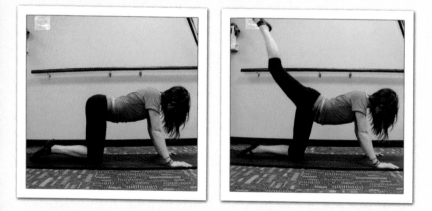

Leg lifts and squats still hold a firm place in my workout routine. I usually incorporate them into the gym routine, if not every time, then usually once a week for maintenance.

I like to alternate movements in my leg lift routine. When one muscle gets too tired I can shift the primary ones being used to secondary use without having to stop using them completely and then I can switch back again.

Place your hands and knees on the ground. Do one leg at a time until failure and then switch to the other leg. Lift your leg in the air as high as you comfortably can, bending the knee slightly as you come up and pointing your foot up to the sky. Do this at least 5 to 10 times before immediately going into the next movement. Next lift your leg to the side, almost like a dog peeing and then kick it out to the side. Yes, I know it's funny, but it works! Do this exercise for the same amount of reps as the other before switching back to the original. I like to do each exercise 2 or 3 times. Start out doing fewer reps before making the switch and slowly build up the amount of time that you can do each movement before switching again.

When doing squats I want you to tap into your "inner ballerina", yes, guys too! You can always do the traditional squats, but I typically do an alternative version that I feel targets the buns a bit more. I like calling them ballerina squats because they feel and look like you're doing a ballet plié.

Be graceful and never fast or forceful. Stand with your feet about a foot apart or more if that's comfortable. Lift up from your heels and stand on the balls of your feet. Bend your knees and go down as far as you can without straining them. Focus your eyes on a single point while you're doing this to help yourself balance. Do this as many times as you are able to. I try to do at least 15. This exercise will help you lift your whole butt as well as strengthen your thighs.

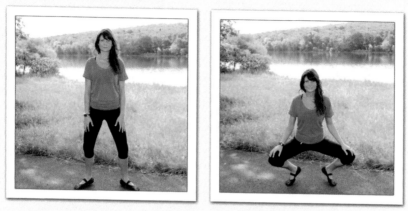

Say Hello to Happy Thighs!

To strengthen and lengthen your thigh muscles without making them look too bulky you want to avoid using heavy weights. Using your own body weight is best. Doing squats, like we covered in the previous section is a great way to tone your quadriceps as well as your butt. Do these 3 times a week to start and once or twice a week for maintenance after that, along with other exercises. There are two other really simple exercises I like to do regularly as well to keep my thighs toned.

Lunges

I like to do lunges without weights and I do one leg at a time as opposed to alternating legs, like they are often done. When I do one leg at a time I get much better results and I don't have to do it as long.

Step one leg back and support yourself with the ball of your foot. Step the other forward and keep it flat on the ground. Have around 2 1/2 feet of space in between your feet, add more or less so that you feel comfortable and can balance properly. Begin slowly bending the knee of your front leg and bend the back leg with it as you dip down. Keep your back straight and your arms pointed down. Only go down as far as you comfortably can or until your knee is at a 90 degree angle. Slowly bring yourself back up again. Start with 5 on each leg and add more as you're able.

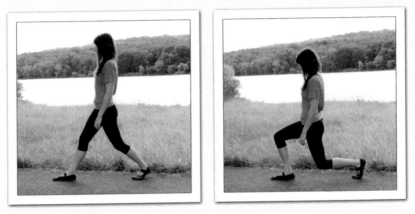

Wall Sit

The next one might look easy but is really hard work. A wall sit is basically what it sounds like, you are putting your back to the wall in a sitting position. Some people modify it and put a large exercise ball in between them and the wall for back comfort and also because you can move up and down if you wanted to make it even harder for yourself.

Put your back up against the wall and slowly start to slide yourself lower, bending your knees. Get as close as you can to bending your knees at a 90 degree angle.

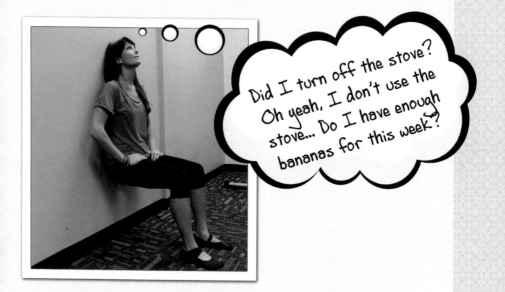

Natural Breast Lift and Chest Toning

A few simple chest exercises can take years off your breasts and create a much more beautiful and full bust line. I noticed a difference after doing them 3 times a week for about 2 weeks.

Chest Press with Free Weights

This exercise will work the pectoral muscles that are going to help lift your chest higher and give you more definition along the top of your chest. They are relatively easy in that you don't need to use heavy weights to see results. I initially used 10 lb. weights and saw good results with them. I have since increased to 15 lb. free weights. Using these size weights are not going to make you bulky, so don't worry about that.

I recommend using an exercise bench for the chest press so that you have proper form. Choose a comfortable weight for you to start out with, 5 or 8 lbs. would be best if it's your first time doing them. Lay flat on your back with your feet on the floor, legs stabilizing you, one on each side of the bench. Hold the free weights at the side of your chest with your arms bent. Slowly bring them up until your arms are straight above your chest. Then bring them back down in the same motion. If you find that you can do it for more than 10 or 15 reps then you might want to try increasing to the next weight up.

If you belong to a gym they may have a machine that does this same motion. I recommend starting with this if you haven't worked out your arms before.

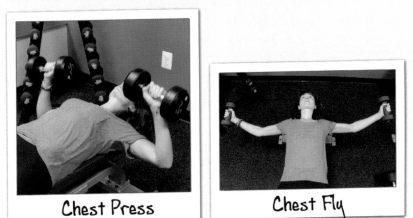

Chest Press

Chest Fly

Chest Fly with Free Weights

This exercise is going to help you tone your chest as well, but it will also focus a little more attention on the underarm area. I know that's a problem area for a lot of people. When I had less muscle tone this used to be a spot I felt self conscious about, and maybe it's not perfect now but it's so much better.

Start out in the same position on the bench as the chest press and use the same weight to begin. Hold your arms up above your chest, but turn your hands inward so the palms are facing each other and bend your wrists in slightly. Keeping your arms almost straight, but bent slightly at the elbows, lower them out to the sides. Feel how far down you'll be able to comfortably go as your arms get closer to becoming parallel with chest. Stop when you're arms are parallel or close to it and go back up. Repeat this around 10 to 15 times.

Pushups

I know, everyone hates pushups and we already covered them, but they are so effective! I just have to give them one more shout out. They will really do wonders for strengthening your chest and many other muscles at the same time. Arms, core, back, legs; you will feel it all.

I try to sneak them in real quick after rock climbing. I usually get to about 10 to 15 after climbing, since I've already had a really good workout.

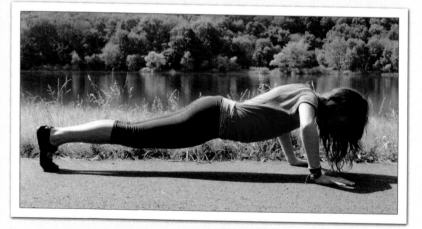

"When Chuck Norris does push ups, he doesn't push up, he pushes the earth down"

Shapely, Toned Arms

Many people use very low weights because they think it will help them avoid getting bulky. You really don't need to worry about that until you start using 20 lb weights or higher for women and maybe 25 lb or higher for men. Start out with whatever weight feels good at first and is not causing you to strain at all. Never sacrifice proper form to use a higher weight before you're ready. A few different arm exercises with free weights can help give your arm a really nice shape.

Bicep Curls

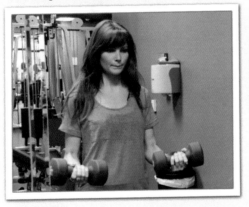

You can see and feel the difference with this exercise rather quickly if you do it 3 times a week. Make sure to choose a weight that is right for your current strength level. When I first started out I used 10 lb weights, then moved to 12.5 lbs three months later. Now I use 15 lb weights. I'm really happy with the shape of my arms right now and I'm not sure if I will ever increase my weight beyond that.

If you can stand in front of a mirror when doing biceps curls it will be a big help at first until you learn what good form feels like. Stand with your back and neck as straight as you can. Keep your feet about a foot apart. Start with the weights down at your sides and slowly bring them up, bending your elbow. Bring them up as far as you comfortably can. Slowly bring them down again until your arm is fully extended. It's important to move at a nice slow pace to avoid swinging your body and straining your neck or shoulders. Aim for 10 to 15 reps or as many as you can do. If you can do more than 20 you might want to try a heavier weight

Upright Row

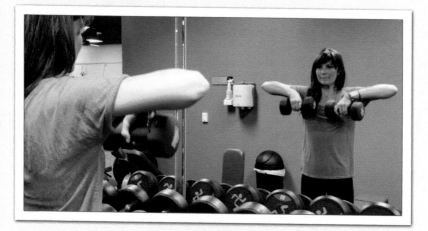

If you want to create a nice shape and flow to your arm then you will want to develop your shoulder or deltoid muscles as well as the biceps and triceps. Doing an upright row can give wonderful results.

Begin in the same starting position as the biceps curl and use the same weight. Turn hands in so your palms are facing you body now instead. Begin to bring the weights up to your chest in the same kind of motion as if you were putting on a pair of pants, except the motion is happening higher on your body.

Keep the weights only about an inch or two away from your body as you to this. Bring your arms down slowly and repeat this exercise 10 to 15 times.

Overhead Tricep Extension

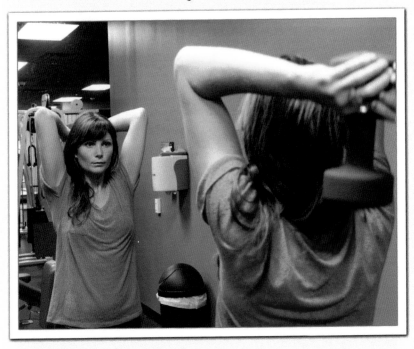

This will really help you feel the burn and tone up your triceps. You may find this exercise more challenging than the others so start out with a slightly lighter weight if you need to. I use a 10 lb. weight for this exercise. We don't usually give them as much attention day to day as the biceps and forearms, so they tend to be weaker.

Stand in the same position as the two previous exercises. Pick out a single free weight that you can comfortably lift above your head. Hold the weight with both hands and lift it straight up over your head. Keeping the upper arm straight up and down, bend your elbow and lower your forearm behind your head. Go as far as you comfortably can and bring the free weight back up.

Wrist Curl

This sounds like a cute little exercise, but it will have you saying, "ooouch!". You want to start with the weight pretty low for this exercise. Some people may choose to sit and rest their arm on a padded bar if they're using a heavier weight and want to focus completely on the forearm. I prefer to do it standing so that I can work the whole arm, still focusing the main attention on the forearm.

Choose a 3 to 5 lb. weight to start with. Hold them in your hands with your palms face down. Raise your arms out in front of you (zombie style!). Then begin to bend your wrist up and down. Do this as many time as you can, but don't overdo it the first time, because the soreness can sneak up on you.

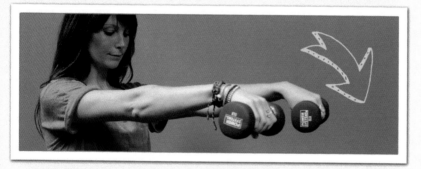

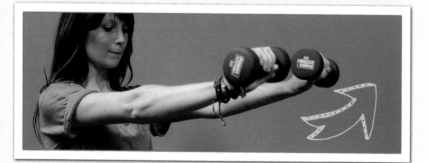

Start Today - Don't Delay!

Most of these workouts can be done at home or without having a gym membership. The exception would be the exercises that require a bench and indoor rock climbing. I hope this section will be helpful to you in creating your own workout routine that suits your needs. If you're trying anything new please consult a doctor first. If you have or are considering a gym membership you may want to do a one-time session with a personal trainer in the beginning to help you achieve proper form for all your exercises.

Staying Motivated to Achieve Your Health and Fitness Goals

1. Write down reasons why you want to achieve your goals, for example: to keep up with my kids; to set a good example for my family; to feel happy with myself and what I have created. Put these reasons where you can see them every day to be reminded of why you do what you do.

2. Set realistic, short term goals so you can see the progress, achieve the goal and set a new one.

3. Make eating healthy and exercising a habit. When you keep it up long enough it becomes a habit, something you just do and don't have to think about. Change your mindset and commit to make it happen. We can accomplish almost anything when we have the right information. Decide to succeed and make it your job to get the information you need to make it happen.

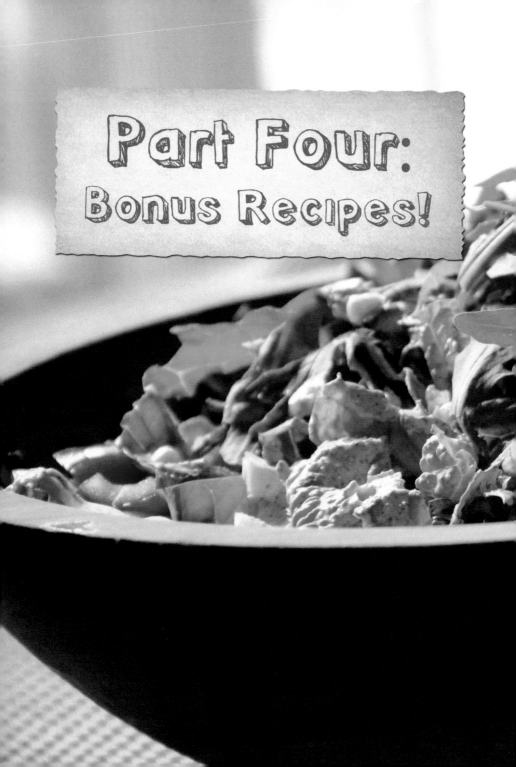

Part Four:
Bonus Recipes!

These recipes are to help you and your family incorporate more raw food into your diet. Hopefully they give you a base to start creating your own delicious raw recipes.

~All recipes serve 1 to 2 people~

Banana Berry Oatmeal Crumble

This recipe is going to keep you full and satisfied well into lunch time. It's the perfect thing to add variety once and while from a fruit mono-meal or a smoothie. (770 calories)

Ingredients:
3 fresh bananas, 3 medjool dates, 1/2 cup of mulberries, 1/2 cup of freeze dried strawberries, 1 tsp of carob powder (raw or toasted), 1/4 tsp of cinnamon

Directions:
Slice the bananas into thin round pieces and place them in a cereal bowl. Chop the fresh dates into quarters. Add the chopped dates, mulberries, strawberries, carob, and cinnamon to the food processor. Pulse them for 30 seconds or until everything looks evenly distributed. Add the berry crumble to the sliced bananas and enjoy!

If you would like this to turn out more like cereal you can blend 1 frozen banana and 2 dates with 1/2 to 1 cup of water and add it to the recipe afterwards. You can subtract the 1 banana and 2 dates from the previous recipe and add it to the banana milk if you would like to keep the calories the same. Otherwise with this addition the recipe comes to 990 calories.

Moo-less Chocolate Raspberry Smoothie

As you can see, this smoothie is even sweet enough for the bees. (750 calories)

Ingredients:
4 bananas, 3 dates, 1 cup raspberry, 4 tbsp raw carob or 2 tbsp toasted carob, 1 coconut (water only, at least 1 1/2 cups), 1/4 tsp vanilla extract

Directions:
Chop the bananas in half or into smaller pieces if you don't have a high speed blender. Put all the ingredients into the blender and blend it until it's smooth.

Cherry Vanilla Ice Cream Sunday

Time travel back to your favorite 50's diner with this yummy treat. (712 calories)

Ingredients:
4 frozen bananas, 3 medjool dates, 1 cup of frozen cherries, 1 tsp of hemp seeds, 1/4 tsp of vanilla extract

Directions:
Chop the bananas into 1 inch slices. Make sure your dates are chopped into quarters as well. Save one of the cherries to put on top of the ice cream. Place all of the ingredients into a high-speed blender or food processor and blend it until the dates and cherries are completely broken up. Scoop the mixture out into a bowl, sprinkle the hemp seeds on top and then add the cherry complete the sundae look!

Megan's Famous Mango Chutney

I first made this easy mango chutney as a chunky salad dressing for myself on my lunch break while working at Arnold's Way. It's so simple to make and it gets devoured at any raw potluck I take it to. (400 calories)

Ingredients:
2 pitted chopped medjool dates, 1 to 2 sliced cucumbers, 2 cups of chopped mango, 2 cups of chopped tomato, 3/4 cup of chopped scallions, 2 tsp of fresh lemon juice

Directions:
Put all the ingredients except the cucumber into a food processor or into a blender with speed control. Pulse chop or blend the mixture on a low speed until it looks like salsa. Put the mixture in a bowl. Surround the edges of a plate with the sliced cucumbers and put the bowl of mango chutney in the center.

Rock'n Ranch Salad

As a kid I saw salad and vegetables as a transporter of ranch dressing. Now I love the taste of vegetables and wouldn't want to drench them in such an unhealthy dressing. I wanted to create a healthy raw version of this classic dressing that wasn't loaded with salt and other junk. This dressing can be put on a salad or used as a veggie dip. (575 calories)

Ingredients:
4 cups of chopped romaine, 2 cups of arugula, 1/2 cup fresh corn, 1/2 cup hemp seed, 1/2 cup fresh chopped scallions, 1/2 cup fresh tomato, 1/4 cup cilantro (not chopped), 2 tbsp of lemon juice, 1/2 tsp fresh dill (not chopped), 1/4 tsp sized piece of fresh rosemary (not chopped)

Directions:
Put the romaine and arugula in a large salad bowl. Put all the other ingredients except the corn and fresh tomatoes in the blender. Blend the mixture until it's creamy and pour it over top over the greens. Add the fresh corn and tomatoes on top of the dressing.

Zucchini Alfredo

Mmmm! You can enjoy this creamy pasta sauce guilt free all by yourself or have a romantic raw meal for two. (690 calories)

Ingredients:
2 large or 4 small zucchinis, 3 leaves of fresh basil, 1 to 2 cups of spinach, 1/2 cup of cashews, 1 cup of sun dried tomatoes, 1/2 cup of chopped fresh tomatoes, 2 tsp of lemon juice, 1/2 tsp of fresh chopped rosemary, 1/4 tsp of fresh thyme, 1/4 tsp of fresh oregano, 1/2 cup of water or more

Directions:
Use a spiral vegetable slicer to spiral the zucchini. I recommend using a thicker cut for this recipe so it's more like fettuccine. Put the zucchini pasta into a large salad bowl and garnish it around the outside with the spinach. Put everything except the fresh tomatoes into the blender. Blend the mixture until it's creamy and add more water as it's needed. Pour the sauce over the zucchini pasta. Add the fresh tomatoes on top for a pop of color and finish it off with some fresh basil leaves.

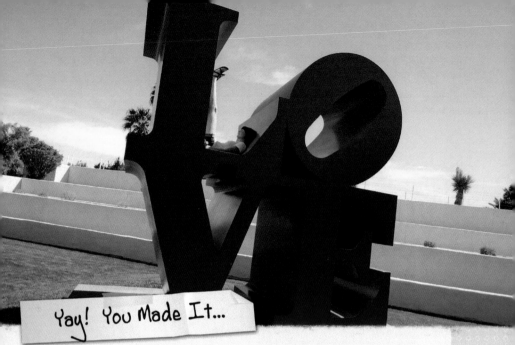

Yay! You Made It...

Everything I've shared with you in this book is from my heart, life experiences, and research. Through my journey with this diet, I've tried to stay true to myself and what I believe while also taking into consideration other points of view.

I have used the knowledge and writings of Dr. Doug Graham and Don Bennett as the base or guideline for my diet. After following their recommendations very closely for many years, I have adapted to it in a way that works for me and I suggest you try the same process to find what is going to satisfy you.

I hope that what I shared is helpful to you on your health journey, wherever you're at, and that you have found the passion and confidence to take responsibility for your own well-being. It may take you one month or many years to get to where you want to be, but the time is going to pass either way so why waste it? 'Someday' is not a day of the week!

Having a strong belief that I am biologically a herbivore and that it is not necessary for me to harm another being for my health is what keeps me on track overall. I think having this as a core belief is very important for many people to stay on track, because our modern society commodifies animals and makes them into no more than a breaded nugget.

We disconnect and forget what we're eating, and we forget that most of us love animals and could not bare to see them suffer the way they currently are, let alone kill them ourselves. We can be easily influenced to forget and 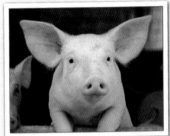 suppress our emotions about what we're eating and it takes a strong compassionate person to take a stand against unnecessary cruelty.

Choosing not to eat animal products is the best change that anyone can make for their own health and for the health of the planet. It is not possible to sustain our planet at the current rate of consumption of animal products. It is destroying our rainforests, oceans, rivers, ozone layer, and air quality more than any other factor or combination of factors.

It may seem overwhelming to try to make a difference in our world today and you may feel like you can't even make a dent. Changing to a vegan diet and lifestyle is the single most effective way to reduce your carbon footprint, save hundreds of thousand of gallons of fresh water per year, save our rainforests, save energy, and reduce damage to the ozone and our air. We only have one planet, so let's act like we actually live on it and keep it beautiful and safe for our children!

Thanks for reading!

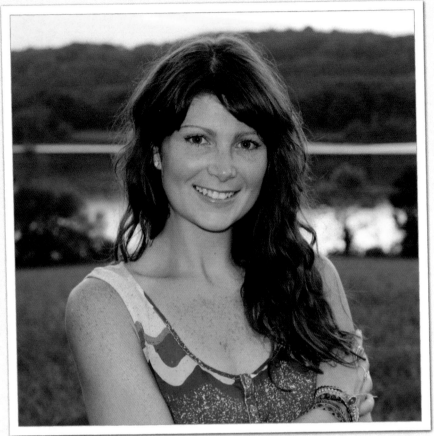

Be sure to check out my website for
free recipes, videos and more fun stuff...

www.MeganElizabeth.com

Made in the USA
Charleston, SC
03 November 2012